The Essential Step-by-Step Guide to
Acupressure
with **Aromatherapy**

Relief for **64** Common Health Conditions

Karin Parramore, LAc, CH

Robert
ROSE

For complete cataloguing information, see page 272.

Disclaimer
This book is a general guide only and should never be a substitute for the skill, knowledge, and experience of a qualified medical professional dealing with the facts, circumstances, and symptoms of a particular case.

The nutritional, medical, and health information presented in this book is based on the research, training, and professional experience of the author, and is true and complete to the best of her knowledge. However, this book is intended only as an informative guide for those wishing to know more about health and medicine; it is not intended to replace or countermand the advice given by the reader's personal physician. Because each person and situation is unique, the author and the publisher urge the reader to check with a qualified health-care professional before using any procedure where there is a question as to its appropriateness. The author and the publisher are not responsible for any adverse effects or consequences resulting from the use of the information in this book. It is the responsibility of the reader to consult a physician or other qualified health-care professional regarding his or her personal care.

Design and Production: PageWave Graphics Inc.
Editor: Fina Scroppo
Copyeditor: Sheila Wawanash
Indexer: Belle Wong
Photographer: Kacey Baxter

Cover
Top Left: Kidney 1 (KI1 • Yongquan), page 54; Top Middle: Dingchuan, page 86; Top Right: Lung 9 (LU9 • Taiyuan), page 26; Bottom: Yintang, page 87.

Additional Images
Cover (bottom): (female) ©iStockphoto.com/&#169 Gansovsky Vladislav; (hand) ©iStockphoto.com/Madiz. Pages 3, 4, 5, 9, 19, 89, 129: (paper background) ©iStockphoto.com/mangpor_2004. Page 8: ©iStockphoto.com/phototake. Page 12: ©iStockphoto.com/roberthyrons. Pages 15, 16, 109 to 127: (paper background) ©iStockphoto.com/tomograf. Page 15: (wood) ©iStockphoto.com/StockImages_AT; (fire) ©iStockphoto.com/saritwuttisan; (earth) ©iStockphoto.com/Tuayai. Page 16: (metal) ©iStockphoto.com/Ensup; (water) ©iStockphoto.com/Mehmet Hilmi Barcin. Page 18: ©iStockphoto.com/simarik. Page 20: ©iStockphoto.com/MarkFGD. Page 88: ©iStockphoto.com/OlgaMiltsova. Page 90: ©iStockphoto.com/MuYeeTing. Page 95: ©iStockphoto.com/SrdjanPav. Page 97: ©iStockphoto.com/skynesher. Page 99: ©iStockphoto.com/simarik. Page 103: ©iStockphoto.com/botamochi. Page 106: ©iStockphoto.com/Catalina-Gabrie Molnar. Page 108: ©iStockphoto.com/toto8888. Page 127: ©iStockphoto.com/Elena Elisseeva. Page 128: ©iStockphoto.com/michelangeloop.

The publisher gratefully acknowledges the financial support of our publishing program by the Government of Canada through the Canada Book Fund.

Published by Robert Rose Inc.
120 Eglinton Avenue East, Suite 800, Toronto, Ontario, Canada M4P 1E2
Tel: (416) 322-6552 Fax: (416) 322-6936
www.robertrose.ca

Printed and bound in Canada

1 2 3 4 5 6 7 8 9 TCP 24 23 22 21 20 19 18 17 16

Contents

Acknowledgments

No book is ever written by the author alone, as I see it. The accumulated influences of every encounter in life are what lead to the concepts embedded in any writing, even if the final words are the author's own. My journey through natural medicine has been so full of amazing people and ideas, I would need another entire book just to thank them all! Instead, I will do what all good authors (and recipients at the Academy Awards) do and thank everyone — all the people who have sparked ideas and explorations, as well as those who accompanied me on my journey. Thank you all.

More specifically, I would like to thank some of the friends who helped me review the technical information, friends I made while attending the National College of Natural Medicine (now the National University of Natural Medicine) in Portland, Oregon, who have remained close to me in so many ways: Dr. Ariel Touchet, Dr. Erick Cervantes, Dr. Brooke Huffman, Dr. Mark Davis (thanks, Mark, for the last three years of learning as well!). Also, my mentors, Dr. Heiner Fruehauf and Brandt Stickley — I promise to write a more classical reference book next time.

Special thanks to Kristine Backes, support gal extraordinaire and dear friend.

I am grateful for the understanding of my landos in Simply Home Community, where I live. They had to endure nearly a year of anxious and grumpy Karin as I learned what it really means to have deadlines and how much hard work goes into writing a book. They were unfailingly understanding, and I love them even more for it.

My mother, Daphne, who stood by to love me in those moments when I was such a cow I couldn't even talk to my landos. Thanks, Mom, for always finding an excuse for my bad behavior. My dad, James R., who stood at my shoulder and whispered words of encouragement, despite being on the other side.

The Portland Threshold Society — despite missing a year of circle, I felt you holding me every step of the way. Mashallah! And thank you. In a similar way, the Thursday morning chanting circle was often the well of calm that helped me through each week.

The writing of this book coincided with so much personal (and global) grief — 2016 will forever be remembered as a year of personal loss. I am deeply grateful for my support group, CoDB, without whom I would likely never have found the reserves to finish this book, and for the support of everyone who held me in my sorrow.

May the strength and determination of dedicated souls be enough.

"Don't deceive with belief." — David Bowie

— Karin Parramore, LAc, CH

Introduction

In this age of technological conveniences, many of us have become removed from a direct connection with nature and its rhythms. Today, many of us live in cities, deep in concrete corridors where even the sun may be only a fleeting visitor.

As technology takes over more of our daily chores, it's no wonder we are not as connected to the cycles of the natural world and rarely rely on our own senses to inform our decisions. We have become so used to "experts" telling us what we should eat, how we should feel, what is an appropriate reaction to world events, among so many other things, that many of us feel at a loss when we are, on rare occasions, required to make these decisions for ourselves.

It does not have to be this way.

We have the ability to choose where we abdicate our responsibility, and where we choose to maintain it. If, for example, we have a traumatic accident, the right decision is to allow medical experts to decide a protocol for our return to health. When it comes to the aggravation of day-to-day symptoms, however, conventional treatments such as drug therapies may not be the best option.

The point is that we have alternatives. Medical systems that have been in place for thousands of years, such as Chinese Medicine, clearly have a lot to offer, especially when we consider that so-called conventional medicine is, to be generous, just a few hundred years old.

If we look more closely at Chinese Medicine, we will see that in ancient times, medical scholars looked to the patterns of nature to understand what health should look like. Then they extrapolated how we, as microcosmic reflections of the macrocosmic big patterns observed in nature, ought to look when maintaining our health.

These patterns, and the channels and acupressure points the ancient practitioners described as a result, are still available for understanding and healing. By learning the course of the channels, and the specific points along them, we can access this information to help reduce symptoms.

This book will help you better understand how the patterns affect our health and how therapies that have a foundation in Chinese Medicine — including acupressure and, more recently, aromatherapy or the use of essential oil blends on acupressure points — can help you take charge of the way you feel on a daily basis, without the use of drugs.

While I have witnessed the modalities of acupressure and aromatherapy to have a dramatic effect on patients, I am not suggesting that these techniques are capable of curing diseases. However, it is primarily the aggravating symptoms of diseases that are problematic on a daily basis. This book offers some ideas for addressing those symptoms in the comfort of one's own home, as often as needed, with a minimum of time and expense. Once the basic techniques (described in Chapters 2 and 4) are understood, acupressure can be applied anytime the symptoms are causing discomfort. With the addition of the essential oil suggestions found in Chapters 3 and 4, the benefits will be even greater.

Please keep in mind that the intent of this book is self-empowerment. You always have the final say in matters of your own health. Any decisions around treatment are ultimately up to the individual, as we learn to pay more attention to our responses and the messages from our bodies. The suggestions given under each condition in Chapter 4 are a great place to start, but this book is intended to encourage further experimentation and learning, from a place of safe, informed curiosity.

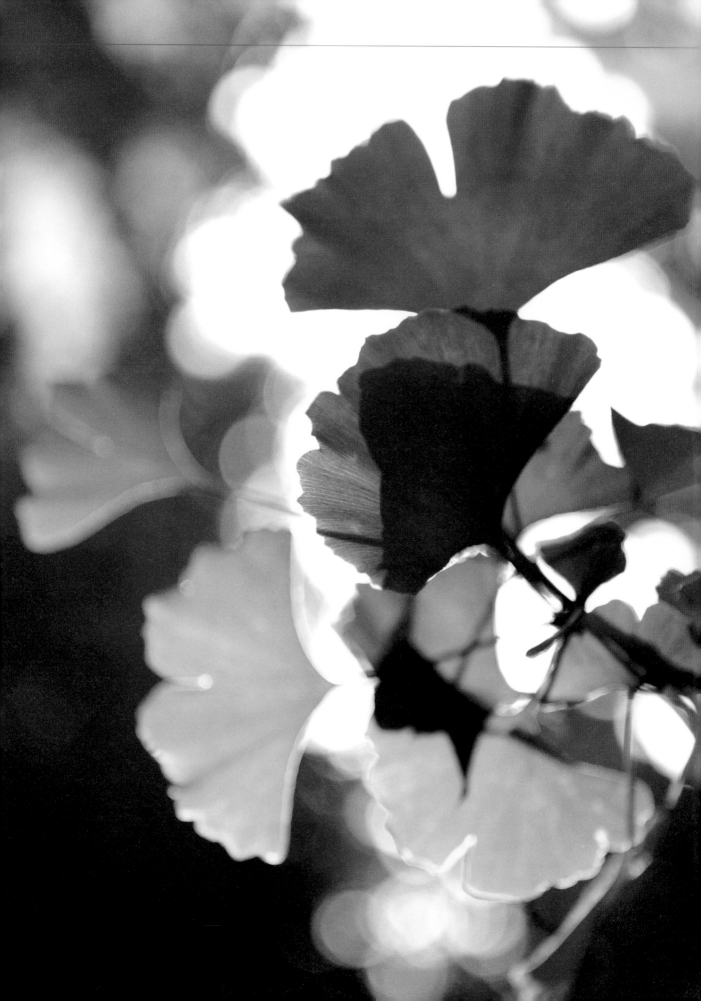

CHAPTER 1

Understanding Chinese Medicine and Its Therapies

What is Chinese Medicine?

The therapies you will find in this book refer specifically to approaches in health and healing that arose in China somewhere between 5,000 and 3,000 years ago. The ancient Chinese scholars were prolific recorders of history, and the concepts that underlie this system of healing were preserved in classical texts like the *YiJing* (also written as *I Ching*), the *Huangdi Neijing (Yellow Emperor's Classic of Medicine)* and the *Shennong Bencao Jing (The Divine Farmer's Classic of Herbal Medicine)*, texts still used by Chinese Medicine practitioners today. What these texts demonstrate is that Chinese Medicine, over thousands of years, developed into a complete, systematic approach to maintaining health.

Connection to Nature

To understand what it means to be a healthy human, the scholars looked to the patterns of nature. Humans (and all living creatures in the material world) were understood to be reflections of larger, more universal patterns that could be "read" through attentive consideration of the world and nature. Seasonal change is a good example. By recognizing the repetitive, cyclic nature of the seasons, we are able to describe a pattern that characterizes that particular time of the year.

The idea is that by taking these universal patterns as models for our lives, we can more easily maintain our health. Not many people would wear a bathing suit outdoors in the winter, for example. We automatically dress warmly without thinking much about it because we know that exposing ourselves to extreme cold will give us a chill, weaken us and, eventually, sap our vitality. While this example may be an obvious one, in truth, all of nature's patterns can inform us about how to stay healthy.

Another good example of how we can live in harmony with nature is the concept of eating locally. Eating foods grown locally is considered by many to be a healthier way to eat, both for us and for our environment, because such goods require less shipping and reduce the carbon footprint. This brings us to another key element of Chinese medicine. The health we try to preserve in this tradition is not just our own personal health, but the health of those around us — our community — as well as the environment.

A Balanced Act

The ancient Chinese understood that we are intimately connected to the land we inhabit, and if it is out of balance, we also become out of balance.

As the ancient scholars observed the world around them for clues, one of the first things they realized was that nothing in nature is static. Rather, the world and its patterns are constantly changing in order to maintain balance. This is a very different approach from modern biological science. Modern biological science usually stops motion of whatever is being observed when testing a theory — the test subject must be stopped and dissected to understand the results. As nothing living ever stops until it dies, the Western approach by definition is often seen more as an examination of death rather than an examination of life.

Diagnosing Health Conditions

Making a diagnosis in Chinese Medicine also reflects this attention to patterns in nature. Diagnostic parameters in essence take a snapshot of the moment in which they are observed. For example, a practitioner might examine the tongue and take a patient's pulse to discern what patterns are playing out in him or her in that moment. If a patient's pulse and tongue are different at the end of a treatment, the regimen is said to have had some affect. Treatments that follow will take these changes into account. There may be a slight modification to the prescription, or the acupuncture treatment may involve different acupoints from those used in the previous treatment.

Modalities of Chinese Medicine

Acupuncture and herbs are the primary modalities of Chinese Medicine, although bodywork therapies, such as shiatsu and tui na, also play a large role. Chinese Medicine's foundational philosophy may be applied to any healing modality; for example, by viewing the essential oils through the lens of Chinese Medicine theory we can gain a richer perspective on their nature and how they can help us address symptoms. Acupuncture involves the insertion of hair-like needles into acupoints — junctions in the body where the qi of the patient can be accessed. The needles act a bit like tiny antennas, connecting to the qi to shift the flow and bring it back into a state of balance. This sounds a bit esoteric and perhaps even magical, but consider similar processes that are more familiar to us, such as the sound of an announcer's voice hitting the ear. We take it for granted, but before the invention of radio, the idea of a device that could transmit sounds over great distances was impossible for most people to imagine.

Qi Connection

Qi is a uniquely Chinese concept that is difficult to define. For our purposes here, we will call it the vital force that flows throughout our body.

In Chinese Medicine, all disease starts at the root, as an imbalance of qi. In a nutshell, the basis of Chinese Medicine thinking can be defined as assessing imbalances in the flow of qi. These imbalances, if left untreated, will eventually lead to other, more overt problems that we label "diseases."

Natural Patterns Disrupted

So what leads to imbalances in the flow? As mentioned earlier, one of the primary causes is not patterning our lives after the larger universal patterns we observe in the rest of nature. As modern life takes us further and further from these patterns, we see greater and more troubling imbalances. Only 150 years ago, people were still dying of epidemics, whereas today we see the rise of slow-brewing, debilitating autoimmune diseases. Our immune system was designed to defend us against naturally occurring invaders — bacteria, viruses or trauma, for example. These days, the signals from our polluted world are generated by substances the body had never experienced in earlier times — plastics, xenoestrogens (synthetic molecules that act like hormones in the body) and the like. These substances are not part of nature and therefore confuse the immune system into attacking its own tissues.

Light pollution is another factor in our move away from natural patterns. When we stay up until 1 a.m. with electric lights blazing, our native sleep cycles are disrupted and the substances that regulate sleep — cortisol and melatonin, for example — become wildly out of alignment. The same can be said of any stimulation late at night, such as working at a computer screen.

Chinese Medicine can help with these conditions, in many cases by reeducating the body about what it is encountering from the outside in order to strengthen communication within it and allow the body's systems to make their own changes. More important, we can educate the patient about how to reconnect with natural cycles. Chinese Medicine practitioners, using acupuncture and herbal medicine, work to bring fluctuating patterns back into alignment with the patterns that we originally followed naturally. While acupuncture and herbs can greatly help, at the root of our treatments we strive to help our patients return to these natural patterns by observing what our patients are eating, how they sleep and, perhaps most important, how they respond to the stress of imbalance.

Yin and Yang

When we say we are "balancing the flow," what we really mean is that we are attempting to correct the interaction between yin and yang. The concept of yin and yang is at the root of Chinese Medicine. Yin and yang are the complementary poles that work together to maintain balance, as all life needs both matter (the more yin aspect) and energy (the more yang aspect) to function. All the classical texts are basically a long survey of everything as seen through the lens of yin and yang, so let's explore these very important terms.

All things in the material world can be defined as containing differing proportions of yin and yang. As doctors, when we take a patient's history, we evaluate if the condition is more yin or yang. If the patient complains, for example, of edema — a condition marked by improper fluid metabolism — we would immediately think, "More yin than yang, because yin represents the more material aspects, such as flesh and fluids, and we are seeing fluid buildup. Still, this is about yang as well, as metabolism, or function, is the yang aspect. Therefore, more yin than yang."

The tendency these days is to see yin and yang as absolutes, to start dividing the world up into this/that: dark is yin, light is yang; male is yang, woman is yin. A better way of stating this would be to say that woman is more yin than man, who is more yang.

In very broad terms, yin is dense matter and yang is diffusive energy. Yin cannot function without yang, and yang cannot be contained without yin to hold it. A living thing in which function and matter are separating is by definition dying.

Ratio of Yin and Yang

Understanding the correct ratio of yin and yang is key to helping maintain balance in all aspects of living, including emotional health. Too much anger, for example, leads to headaches and heart disease, as the yang is constantly rising up with each bout of rage. We would balance that by drawing the yang back down out of the upper part of the body, to start. To give a more physical example, if a patient complains of watery diarrhea, we would diagnose that as not having enough yang to properly digest food. We would treat this by encouraging an increase of digestive yang, or a movement of yang inward, toward the center where digestion takes place.

No Absolutes

In the material world, nothing is pure yin or pure yang; by definition, any material object is a blending of the two and living matter is impossible without this blending.

Greater Patterns

When we move beyond the (seeming) duality of yin and yang, it quickly becomes apparent that nature is easily divided into larger patterns as well. Throughout time and across all human experiences, these same ideas have been explored, of course, because they are so basic to life, but each tradition saw the divisions of nature slightly differently. In the European and Western Asian tradition, for example, the four elements were understood as earth, air, fire and water. In China, the idea developed into five elements — wood, fire, earth, metal and water. (It is interesting that air is not seen as a separate category; in Chinese philosophy, wind, or air, is most closely allied with wood, for we "see" invisible air when the trees sway.)

The Five Elements

The five-element system, like the idea of yin and yang, is crucial to Chinese Medicine. It is one of the earliest systems for categorizing the material world more specifically and is used extensively in the *Huangdi Neijing*, one of the early medical classics of ancient China. Combining the ideas of yin and yang with five elements further refines and clarifies the qualities of yin and yang in specific instances. While the five elements are easy to understand as elements alone, the same characteristics we ascribe to them can be used to understand human physiology and pathology. Fire, for example, by its very nature is yang — it is hot, it moves, it is necessary to maintain life. We see the metabolic processes of the body as fire-like. Digestion is understood to be a type of "cooking" within the body that liberates the nutrients in the foods we eat. If we apply the thinking behind yin and yang onto five elements, we see that yang fire implies doubled fire — yang is diffusive energy and enables metabolism — and brings to mind a roaring bonfire that can easily get out of control. This could be at the root of a condition like acid reflux, for example — a digestive fire grown out of control. (See GERD/Acid Reflux, page 192, for more information.)

To apply the same idea to another element, yang wood is like new green grass, vigorously growing, changing every day, easily renewing itself when mowed. That bright, clear green of new grass feels more vital than that of a tree, where most of the action is on the inside — trees would be described as yin wood. Like fire, wood is more yang than yin — the movement of wood qi is up and out and yang goes up — but less yang than fire because wood is tethered to the earth. Wood grows out of the earth, so it cannot ascend as high as fire can, which makes it less yang than fire. Once a fire no longer has a fuel source, it dies down, with small sparks flying off for hours until all the heat is gone. To relate this to the body, when we start to lose our yang fire, we are approaching the end of our life.

The qualities of each element are assigned to all aspects of being alive, material as well as physiological functions. Wood, for example, is flexible. As noted above, it has a gesture of up primarily, but also out, yet it is also rooted. Anything occurring in nature that moves up from a rooted place will have some association with wood, although the association may not be immediately apparent. Fighting for one's beliefs even in the face of opposition, for example, is a wood quality.

The opposite is also true — inflexibility in any capacity can be viewed as a wood pathology, also described as a lack of the essential quality of wood. If someone is experiencing inflexibility in their life, working with acupoints on the wood channels (liver and gallbladder points) with essential oils that support or soften this quality (rose geranium, for example) can be very effective.

Disease = Imbalance

Chinese Medicine theory recognizes that most symptoms of disease are the body's attempt to bring itself back into balance. Disease is recognized as a part of oneself, and not an enemy to be conquered.

To gain a deeper understanding of the five elements, let's explore some of the qualities associated with each. Keep in mind that these qualities can be described as physiologically appropriate or pathologically imbalanced. A pathology is basically anything that manifests as the opposite of the physiologically appropriate qualities. First, however, it is important to note that physiological balance exists on a spectrum with pathological manifestations; if balance lies at the center point, then pathologies can be anywhere else on the spectrum.

Stubborn, inflexible attachment to a goal, for example, might be at one end, while the inability to focus enough to work toward a goal might be at the other end. The modalities offered in this book help us stay closer to the center point.

Five Elements of Chinese Medicine
Essential concepts of each element

WOOD

Gesture
(the direction in which the energy, or qi, tends to move)

Up and out

Physiologically Appropriate Qualities

Goal-oriented • Flexible • Vigorous • Promotes growth • Enthusiastic • Compassionate • Can be righteously angry • Shows leadership • Pushes against gravity (think trees) — moves blood up through the system • Keeps tendons healthy (wood governs all string-like structures in the body, such as tendons, nerves, hair and nails)

Pathologies
Pathological gesture: **collapsing down and in**

Inflexibility or overly flexible (both emotionally and physically) • Narrow-mindedness (overly goal-oriented) or inability to set goals • Stunted or reckless growth • Inability to rise when help is needed or exhaustion due to agreeing to everything • Undirected anger or the courage of your convictions • Blood stagnation • Tendon weakness

FIRE

Gesture
(the direction in which the energy, or qi, tends to move)

Like wood, still up and out, but more expansive, less single-minded. Fire can rapidly change direction, unlike wood, which tends to move more slowly

Physiologically Appropriate Qualities

Yang fire is both the central core and the physiological functions that take place at the periphery of the body: maintaining a core temperature is one end and keeping the extremities warm is the other • Devoted — imagine the glow when one is gazing upon a loved one • Warm • Enthusiastic bursts of creativity or intuition, like flames dancing in a fire • Maintains healthy blood flow and vessels (with wood energy) • Keeps heart — both the emotional and physiological heart — healthy

Pathologies
Pathological gesture: **"burning out," flying up and away or unable to raise the fire**

Restlessness or ennui • Insomnia or hypersomnia • Mania followed by depression • Headaches, edema of the feet • High blood pressure or chronically low blood pressure

EARTH

Gesture
(the direction in which the energy, or qi, tends to move)

Lemniscate, which is the ability to go out into the world, experience it and bring it back to center for processing on a personal level — all while maintaining groundedness

Physiologically Appropriate Qualities

Dynamically stable — able to remain centered in an ever-changing environment; grounded, but in the way a dancer is, or a sailor on a ship • Centered • Nurturing • Generous • Satisfied with enough for whatever is needed, whoever needs it • Maintains good digestion

Pathologies
Pathological gesture: **no movement, stuck in the mud, spinning tires**

Stuckness (material, emotional, mental, environmental) or inconsistency • Laziness or tendency to be driven solely by other's ideas or desires • Greediness or carelessness with resources • Inability to nourish others or sycophantism (being completely self-serving) • Tendency to overeat or inability to eat many things • Digestive problems

METAL

Gesture
(the direction in which the energy, or qi, tends to move)
Descending — metal falls; it is the sword that cuts away the unnecessary

Physiologically Appropriate Qualities
Healthy elimination • Healthy respiration • Upright in character • Uses ritual as a centering practice and a way to connect to spirit • Structured • Respectful • Willing to make hard decisions and cut away the unnecessary

Pathologies
Pathological gesture:
rigid or too much descent — freefall
Rigidity, both of mind and body • A tendency to be judgmental or naive • A tendency to be dogmatic or easily swayed • A tendency to be obsessive or easily swayed • A tendency to be a bully or timid • Weak lung qi • Constipation

WATER

Gesture
(the direction in which the energy, or qi, tends to move)
Go low; completely descended, as in an obeisance or bowing

Physiologically Appropriate Qualities
Humble • Reserved • Deeply respectful of the source of life • Willing to step aside in favor of another • Able to work under another's authority • Healthy urination and fluid metabolism • Strong bones • Strong, flexible spine

Pathologies
Pathological gesture:
frozen, inability to descend
Hubris (excessive or unfounded sense of self-worth) or spinelessness • Reclusivity or excessively open • Lack of respect for spiritual matters or mindless devotion • Inability to listen to another's opinion or inability to form one's own opinion • Stiff-necked • Problems with urination, water metabolism • Bone diseases • Spine problems

Channel Theory

The final key concept of Chinese Medicine is channel theory. Channels are described as the places where the qi, vital energy, flows through the body; that is, the riverways that move vitality to all corners of the body. For acupressure, we use acupuncture points to reach these riverways of vitality.

To speak metaphorically, acupuncture points (acupoints) on the channels can be compared to regions along a river. For example, at junctions of the body with similar features (such as ankles and wrists), the acupoints often have parallel functions, in much the same way that the ports of rivers always occur where the river is wide, deep and calm. Rivers are used to move resources and we want that to occur as seamlessly as possible, at the safest point along the river. It does not make sense to have a port at some rapids, an area defined by fierce and often unpredictable or surprising movement — that region is obviously better for moving swiftly.

Junction Points

To return to the points on the body, the different locations around junctions such as ankles and wrists relate to the different channels. If one is trying to access resources specifically for the kidney channel, for example, the point of choice would be Kidney 3, right behind the inner ankle bone (see page 55). This place on the body was determined by the ancient Chinese Medicine practitioners to be like a good site for a river port — wide, deep and calm, and thus able to easily offer resources. There are also acupoints clustered at areas that are more like oceans, vast and placid, excellent at receiving the rivers and draining fluids from the land (many of these points are around the elbows and knees). If the need is to rapidly change a symptom like fever, for example, it is better to press points that are more like the rapids. These points are often found at the ends of the fingers and are chosen based upon where the fever is occurring (or in which channel).

Adding Essential Oils

So if we think of the channels as rivers, and the points as different ports with different features, the concept of treating the points with minute quantities of essential oils (in the manner described in Chapter 4: "Acupressure and Aromatherapy For Conditions") makes more sense. Essential oils are able, in a way, to take the place of the needles and act as an antenna, as they easily enter the body through the skin. Specifically, applying them to the suggested points is even more helpful — we can access the qi at any point, but we choose the ports that make the most sense. Why go to the ocean if you want to find the rapids? Perhaps we need to slowly influence a system, gently reshape it to allow smooth flow. Small adjustments to the banks of a river over time will result in the riverbed taking a new direction. If we tried to change that riverbed by brute force, the entire ecosystem could collapse. If we apply this idea to the body, perhaps the "riverbed" has narrowed due to atherosclerosis, or plaque in the arteries. The very last thing we would want to do is tear away at the plaque, because this could lead to an embolism. Instead, through a combination of essential oils and acupoints, we work to gently dissolve the plaque into amounts the body can safely process. On the other hand, there are times — such as emergency situations — when fast change is necessary. Being able to dive deep and open a space for the flow can, in some cases, immediately reduce pain.

Harmony and Balance

In this chapter, the major concepts of Chinese Medicine have been briefly outlined to offer a bit of background to the systems offered elsewhere in this book and with the hope that this short explanation may help readers understand why it works and how this practice can help return us to balance. Harmony and balance are all-important to Chinese Medicine. It is easier to compensate for small changes more often than to try to restore a body that has swung wildly out of balance. Regular use of the techniques described in this book can go a long way to maintaining our native resources and enhancing health.

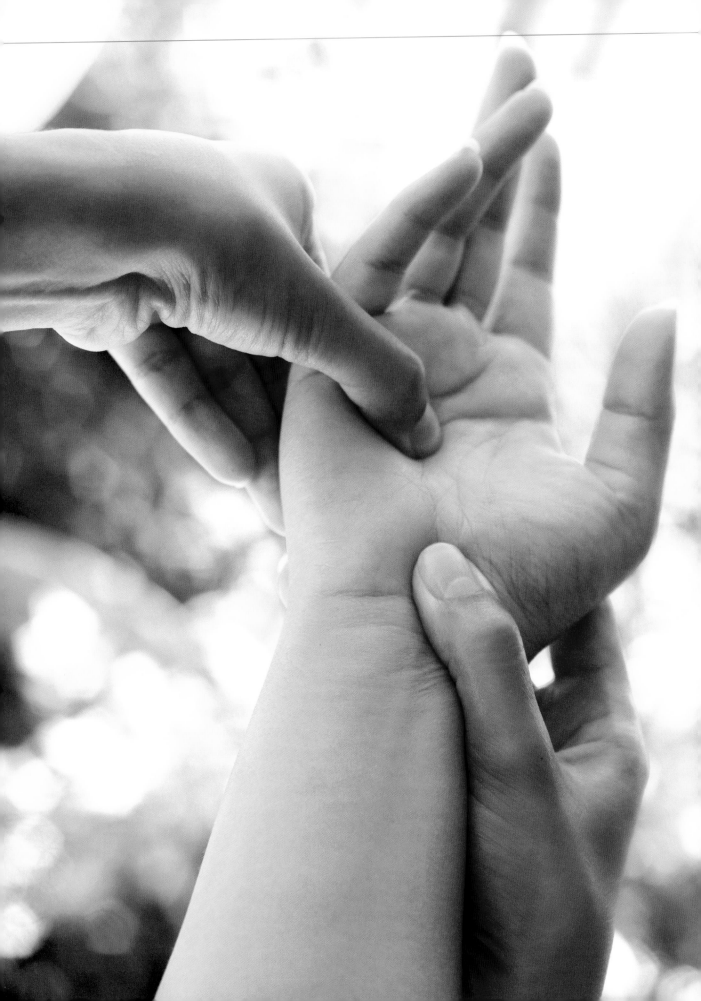

CHAPTER 2

Acupressure Points

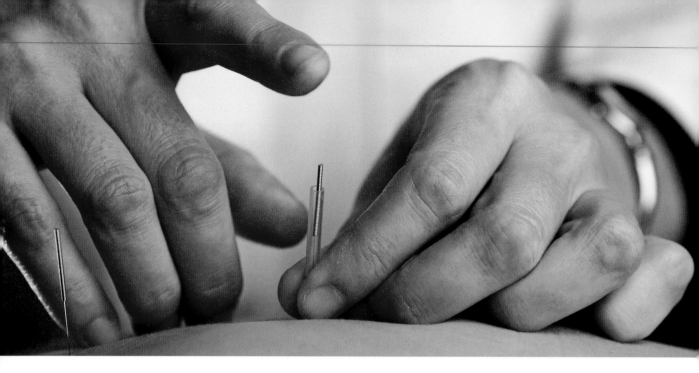

Acupressure vs. Acupuncture

Acupressure is based on acupuncture, a treatment in which filiform (hair-like) needles are inserted into acupuncture points (acupoints) to stimulate a number of different responses. From a purely biomedical perspective, acupuncture is known to stimulate the immune response that occurs at anytime we insert something foreign into the body. There may be changes in the tissues at the site of the insertion, among other things. Hormonal changes can take place, for example, leading to a sense of calm and relaxation. From a Chinese Medicine perspective, the needle is a conduit for the qi (energy, or life force) in the universe to interact with the qi of both the practitioner and the patient. As described in the chapter on Chinese Medicine (see Chapter 1), the patterns of nature guide the patterns within our bodies, and sometimes we need to reconnect with those universal blueprints to maintain a sense of well-being.

As an acupuncturist, I can sense changes in the patterns and I work with patients to help smooth the flow of qi. Most times, I am working to remove blockages and encourage qi to return to those places in the body where it is deficient, in order to restore order to the system; in other words, such treatments help the body remember the pattern of health by removing the blocks to health. There are several tools that assist with this process — needling, massage, herbs and essential oils, for example. In most cases, it takes many years to attain both proficiency at needling and a license to practice acupuncture. For practitioners attempting to work with the root pattern, it makes sense that we would need a great deal of training. The ability to address the symptoms, however, is something everyone should be able to achieve. Reducing discomfort or improving digestion, for example, can greatly improve the quality of life as we work through the process of returning the body to a place of balance.

As mentioned, simply pressing on the acupoint with the intention of smoothing the imbalances can be remarkably effective. With the addition of essential oils to the treatment, we take advantage of the temperature, nature and direction of the oil to further adjust the imbalances of qi. Temperature refers to the influence of the oil on the body, while direction influences whether the qi will move up, down or circulate. Applying essential oil dilutions to an acupoint before pressing allows the chemical compounds, and their message of change, to enter the channel at the places best suited for correcting change, and these are the points Chinese medical practitioners have been using for thousands of years. Channels are the rivers of movement in the body, along which qi (vital force) travels. In other words, the oils may be able to function in place of the needles. (See Chapters 3 and 4 for more information.)

Before Treatment

For the best results, it is important to make time and space for the treatment — try to perform the acupressure when you can focus, in a place where you will not be disturbed or distracted, especially when first learning the technique.

Before you begin applying the treatment, get a sense of where the points are located on the body. You can learn to do this through sensing tissue changes. This is much easier to experience than most people think. Start by gently palpating — touching mostly with the fingertips — along the lines of the channels to see if you can feel the energy pathway. With practice, you will gain a sense of the course it runs. Next, use the detailed, step-by-step instructions listed throughout this chapter to precisely locate the acupressure points.

Locating the Acupressure Points

Fortunately, many of the acupressure points (acupoints) exist over naturally occurring dips and depressions on the body, and the finger will fall into these quite naturally when palpating.

Applying Pressure

Once the point has been confidently located, it is time to apply the pressure. It is not necessary to apply very much pressure. In fact, firm and steady is more important than really deep pressure. The tissue should not be pressed to the point of frank pain, although it may well be sensitive or uncomfortable (this is often a sign you are on the right track!). If there is an indentation of the tissue that remains for more than 10 seconds after removing your finger, reduce the pressure a bit at the next point. There should *never* be bruising.

On the other hand, the pressure applied needs to be great enough to easily feel the sensation. Most importantly, pay attention to your body's feedback. Is there an increase in pain or discomfort when you press a point? It may be that the imbalance is resolving, or it may mean you need to lessen the pressure. The more you learn to listen to the feedback, the easier it will become to gauge what your body is telling you.

Achieving Balance

Most of the points are bilateral; that is, the points are matched on each side of the body. For most conditions, pressing both points is a good idea — remember, the body is an interdependent system and any influence your treatment exerts will affect the whole body. Balancing will likely happen faster if both sides are equally addressed. If possible, first find and then press both sides at the same time. The exception is the points on the front of the neck — ST9, for example, where it is possible to block both of the major arteries leading to the head. Doing this will lead to unconsciousness, just like in the movies! Exercise *caution* when you use ST9, and always press one side after the other.

If the condition is one-sided, it may be easier to treat the points on the opposite side, especially if a suggested point is close to an area of pain or discomfort. This may seem odd, but because the two sides of the body are basically a mirror image, treating the opposite side will benefit the side with the pain or injury, for a fascinating reason that is beyond the scope of this book.

Accessing Acupressure Points

It is often necessary to maintain tension in certain parts of the body to access the points on your own. For example, to treat foot points requires bending over, and to access the neck points may require holding the arms up for an extended period, which many people find uncomfortable. It is important to find the most comfortable position for accessing the points so they can be pressed for an adequate amount of time without leading to discomfort. You will find suggestions for positioning in each acupoint description to help achieve the greatest ease.

The points described here were chosen first for their function, but accessibility was also a key consideration. Self-treatment requires a person to be able to reach the point easily. It may be easier, however, to enlist the help of another individual to access some of the points. If someone is assisting, be sure to direct them precisely on where the point is located. Communicate clearly about your responses and give good verbal feedback so the helper does not press too hard, for example.

How Often Can I Use Acupressure?

The points can be pressed many times throughout the day, as desired. As long as the guidelines around pressure are followed, it is difficult, for the most part, to overtreat with acupressure. Again, listen to the feedback from your body. Be sure to also drink a large glass of water following an acupressure treatment.

Using Essential Oils On Acupressure Points

The use and frequency of essential oil blends on acupoints does have some limitations. Suggestions for their application and how they are used with acupoint treatments are found in Chapter 4: "Acupressure and Aromatherapy for Conditions." The recommended dilutions (found in the chart starting on page 109) are deemed the safest way to use them: overuse can lead to problems. Sensitization of the skin is most commonly caused by oxidized oils (see page 102) but has been known to occur if the oils are used too frequently. Although this is fairly rare, it can still occur.

At the recommended dilutions, a safe maximum use is three to four times a day for no longer than 7 days. If the area still requires further treatment, create a new protocol, something quite easy to do since there are multiple points and oils suggested under each condition. Additionally, other treatments found on each condition page in Chapter 4 can strategically support an acupressure protocol.

Varying Times

The length of time to hold each point is also dependent on personal experience. Some people hold for shorter periods of time but repeat the pressure several times in one treatment. Others suggest holding the point for a set amount of time — for example, 30 seconds to a minute — but these are mostly arbitrary guidelines. We are pressing to smooth the flow of qi and when this starts to happen, it can easily be felt when we learn to listen to our bodies.

When you first begin, start by holding the point for about 30 seconds, then break to see if there is a change — less pain, increased ease in the tissue, for example — before pressing for another 30 seconds. Repeat up to three times in a session.

As always with any treatment, if any unexpected side effects occur, stop pressing. Side effects may include headache, dizziness, nausea or emotional flares. Many people are very responsive to acupressure and do not expect an immediate result even though it's quite normal.

Finally, always try to give yourself at least a minute or two to integrate the changes before leaving the "treatment space." This allows the body to retain the benefits for a longer period of time.

Selecting Acupressure Points

Each acupoint helps specific conditions. Review the boxes titled "Helps With These Conditions," as well as Chapter 4, to determine how and when to apply certain acupressure point treatments.

Lung 1

This point is located on the upper lateral chest (furthest from the center), near the arm.

Helps with these conditions

- coughs of all kinds
- heat in the chest
- sore throat
- asthma, especially with accessory muscle involvement
- fever
- chills

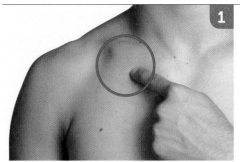

1 To locate the point, stand in front of a mirror to view the upper chest. Locate the clavicle (collarbone).

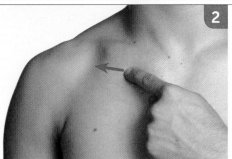

2 Slide the tip of the index finger along the bottom of the collarbone toward the arm until it lands on a deep depression just before the swell of the deltoid muscle on the front of the arm.

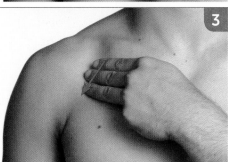

3 Next, slide the finger three-fingers width down the chest and along the curve of the deltoid, until the finger lands on a depression.

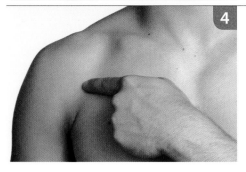

4 Where the finger lands on the center of this depression is where you will find the point.

Lung 7

This point is located on the crest of the forearm, very close to the wrist.

Helps with these conditions			
• common cold	• sore throat	• adhesive	• asthma
• sneezing	• stiff neck	capsulitis	• bronchitis
• runny nose	• headache	(frozen shoulder)	

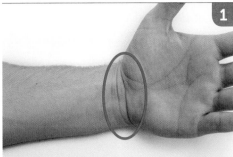

1 To locate the point, rest the hand on a comfortable surface, palm side facing up. Locate the wrist crease by slightly bending the hand up. Relax the hand.

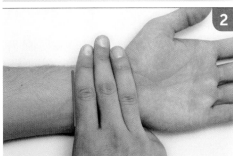

2 With your other hand, lay the three middle fingers horizontally along the crease, with the fourth (ring) finger positioned on the crease itself.

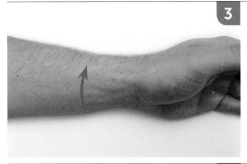

3 Next, roll the tip of the index finger up and over the radius bone, the bone on the thumb side of the forearm.

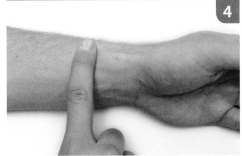

4 Where the tip of the finger lands on the radius bone is where you will find the point.

Lung 9

This point is located on the wrist.

Helps with these conditions

- Raynaud syndrome
- cough
- wheeze
- phlegm
- belching
- excessive yawning
- weak lung function

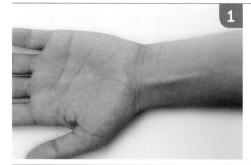

1 To locate the point, rest the hand on a comfortable surface, palm side facing up.

2 Locate the wrist crease by slightly bending the hand up. Relax the hand.

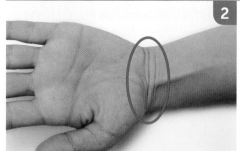

3 Next, slide the tip of the index finger from your opposite hand along the wrist crease toward the space under the thumb until it lands on a large depression.

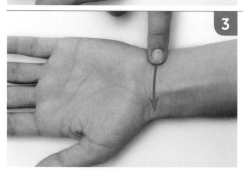

4 Where the index finger rests on this depression is where you will find the point.

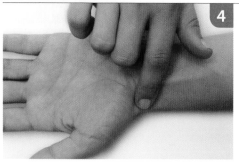

Lung 10

This point is located on the palm of the hand, on the thenar eminence (the fleshy base of the thumb).

Helps with these conditions

- hiccups
- shortness of breath
- painful cough

- heat and dryness in the chest, nose, throat or lungs

- sore throat
- dry throat

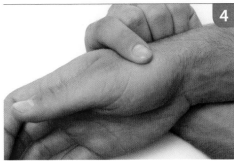

1 To locate the point, find the thenar eminence on the palm of the hand, the fleshy mound at the base of the thumb.

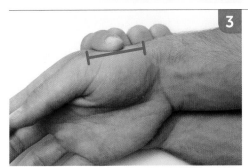

2 Locate the metacarpal bone of the thumb (the bone that connects the thumb to the wrist) that defines the lower edge of the fleshy mound and is found in between the first joint of the thumb and the wrist.

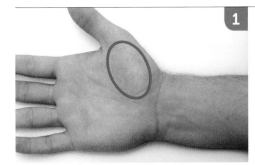

3 Next, slide the tip of the index finger along the metacarpal bone to the midway of the bone, approximately halfway between the wrist and the first joint of the thumb.

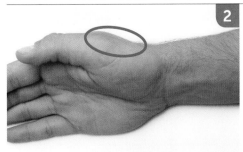

4 The point is located between the bone and the muscles that make up the thenar eminence. Slide the finger over the curve of the bone. Where the finger lands on the space between the bone and the muscles of the mound is where you will find the point.

Lung 11

This point is located on the thumb, near the nail.

Helps with these conditions

- epicondylitis (tennis elbow, golfer's elbow)
- sore throat
- dry throat
- nosebleeds
- fever in children, especially with childhood diseases

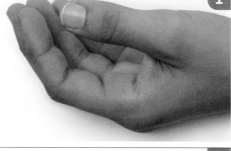

1 To locate the point, rest the hand on a comfortable surface, palm side facing up, ensuring thumb is elevated.

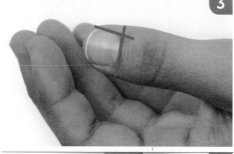

2 Note the line along the bottom of the thumb nail.

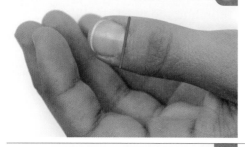

3 Note another line along the lateral (outer) edge of the nail, the edge farthest from the index finger.

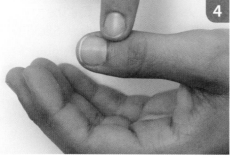

4 Where these two location lines intersect is where you will find the point.

Large Intestine 4

This point is located on the dorsal (back) side of the hand, near the base of the thumb.
Warning: Avoid during pregnancy — can cause contractions.

Helps with these conditions

• the first signs of a cold or flu	• red or hot eyes	• mouth sores	• bacterial infections
• headache	• nosebleed	• sore throat	• may speed delivery in childbirth
	• toothache	• tinnitus	

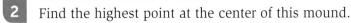

1 To locate the point, move the thumb toward the index finger until the two are pressed together. This will cause a fleshy mound of skin to bunch up on the back of the hand, between the index finger and thumb.

---

2 Find the highest point at the center of this mound.

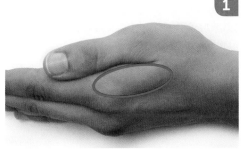

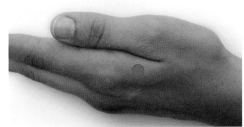

3 Where the finger lands on the center of this high point is where you will find the point.

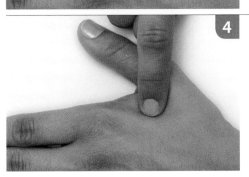

4 Be sure to relax the thumb before pressing the point.

Large Intestine 5

This point is located on the dorsal (back) side of the hand, close to the wrist.

Helps with these conditions

- frontal headache
- toothache
- any condition of the face and sensory organs

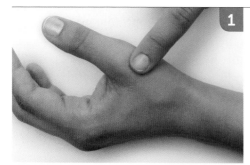

1 To locate the point, place the index finger from the opposite hand on the metacarpal bone (the bone that connects the thumb to the wrist).

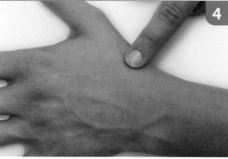

2 Slide the finger down the thumb bone toward the wrist on the dorsal (back) side of the hand until the tip of the finger rolls off the end of the bone and lands on a depression, just before hitting the wrist bone.

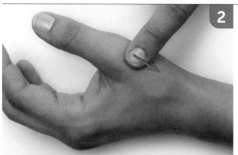

3 To confirm the location of the point, alternatively, spread all the fingers and thumb widely to engage all the tendons in the hand. The anatomical snuffbox (an obvious triangular-shaped dip made up of the two thumb tendons and the wrist) will appear on the back of the hand below the thumb.

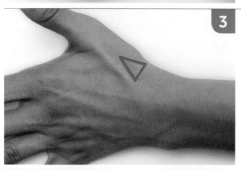

4 In the center of this dip is where you will find the point.

Large Intestine 11

This point is located on the forearm, very close to the elbow.

Helps with these conditions

- atopic dermatitis (eczema)
- acne
- any condition of the skin
- fever
- viral infections

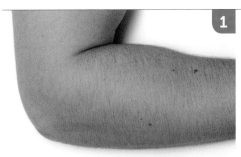

1 To locate the point, bend the arm 90 degrees.

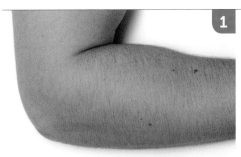

2 With the tip of the index finger from the opposite hand, locate the lateral (outermost) end of the elbow crease.

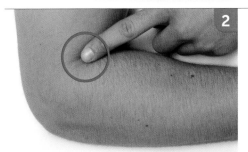

3 Next, slide the finger laterally (away from the body) three fingers' width toward the elbow bone to locate the olecranon process of the elbow, the bony prominence closest to the elbow crease.

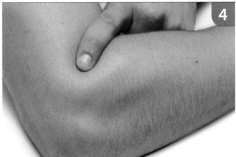

4 Where the finger lands on the midpoint between the elbow crease and the olecranon process is where you will find the point.

Large Intestine 15

This point is located on the anterior (front) of the shoulder.

Helps with these conditions

- adhesive capsulitis (frozen shoulder), especially at the anterior (front) of the shoulder
- any imbalance of the shoulder

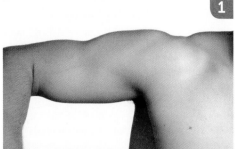

1 To locate the point, stand in front of a mirror. Bend the arm 90 degrees and raise the elbow until it is level with the shoulder.

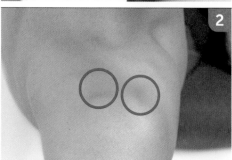

2 This will cause two depressions to appear next to each other at the top of the shoulder. If they are not obvious, palpate for them just above the deltoid muscle at the top of the arm.

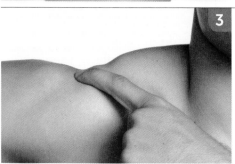

3 Next, use the index finger from the opposite hand to find the depression that is in the anterior (front).

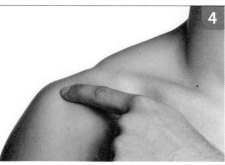

4 Where the finger lands on the depression closest to the chest is where you will find the point. Be sure to relax the arm before pressing the point.

Large Intestine 20

This point is located on the face, very close to the nose.

Helps with these conditions

- any condition of the nose
- nasal congestion
- nosebleed
- rhinitis (runny or stuffy nose)
- sneezing
- anosmia (loss of sense of smell)

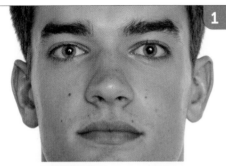

1 To locate the point, look at your face in a mirror.

2 Place the tip of the index finger in the nasolabial groove, the area between the outer edge of the nostril and the upper lip.

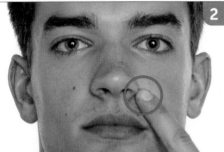

3 It may help to smile when locating the groove.

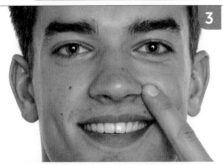

4 Where the finger falls at the top of the groove, closest to the nostril, is where you will find the point.

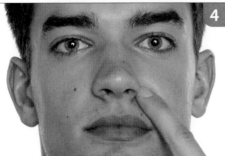

Stomach 6

This point is located on the lower jaw.

Helps with these conditions

- toothache in the lower jaw
- temporomandibular joint (TMJ) pain
- gum disease
- deviation of the mouth after a stroke

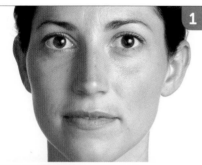

1 To locate the point, look at your face in a mirror.

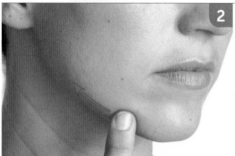

2 Gently clench the teeth and slide an index finger along the lower jawbone from the chin toward the back of the jaw until it finds the mound slightly above the jawbone.

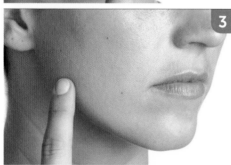

3 To ensure the correct location of the mound, relax the jaw and the mound will disappear.

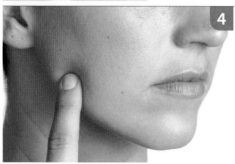

4 The direct center of this mound is where you will find the point.

Stomach 7

This point is located on the jaw.

Helps with these conditions

- skin blemishes (acne)
- deafness, tinnitus, ear pain
- toothache of the upper jaw

- muscle spasms of the face
- trigeminal neuralgia
  (facial nerve pain)

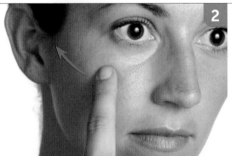

1 To locate the point, look at your face in a mirror.

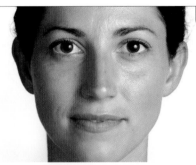

2 Locate the top of the zygomatic arch (cheekbone) and slide an index finger along the outer edge of it toward the ear until it runs into the joint of the jaw. To test that the finger is at the joint, open the mouth wide — it should feel as though the jawbone is pushing the finger out of the depression.

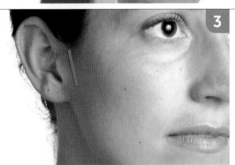

3 The fingertip should be in a depression about one thumb's width from the tragus, the small flap of cartilage at the front of the ear.

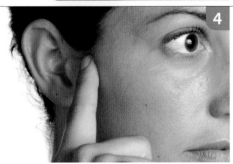

4 The direct center of this depression is where you will find the point.

Stomach 8

This point is located on the head at the upper corners of the face, just inside the hairline.

Helps with these conditions		
• alopecia (hair loss) • frontal headache • splitting headache	• excessive eye tearing, especially with outdoor activity	• one-sided facial paralysis

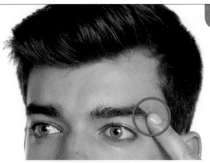

1 To locate the point, look at your face in a mirror. With the tip of the index finger, find the outer end of the eyebrow.

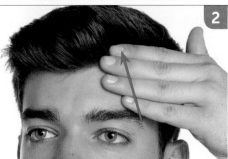

2 Slide the index finger straight up from the inner temple (the part of the temple closest to the end of the eyebrow) until the finger is about four fingers' width above the eyebrow.

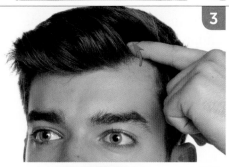

3 Next, note the divot at the hairline, then extend the index finger into the hairline about another half an inch (1 cm) beyond the divot to the slight depression further back on the head.

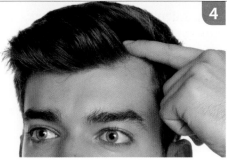

4 Where the finger lands on the center of this depression is where you will find the point.

Stomach 9

This point is located on the throat, level with the highest point of the laryngeal prominence (Adam's apple).

Helps with these conditions

- thyroid imbalance
- any condition of the throat
- dizziness
- feelings of dissociation

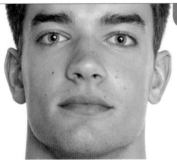

1 To locate the point, look at your face in a mirror.

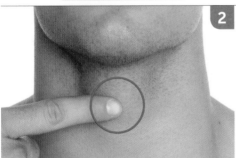

2 Locate the laryngeal prominence and find the high point.

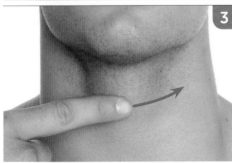

3 Next, slide an index finger laterally (to either side of the point) until the finger tip encounters the sternocleidomastoid, the large muscle about three fingers' width from the high point of the Adam's apple.

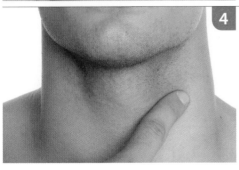

4 Where the finger falls at the medial (inner) border of this muscle, the edge closest to the Adam's apple, is where you will find the point.

Stomach 25

This point is located on the abdomen, at the level of the umbilicus (belly button).

Warning: Avoid during pregnancy — may cause too much pressure on the baby.

Helps with these conditions

- constipation
- all intestinal imbalances

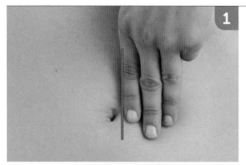

1 To locate the point, lie down and expose the lower abdomen. Locate the umbilicus. Place three fingers vertically (fingertips pointing down) against the lower abdomen, measured from the belly button, so that the edge of the index finger is against the outer edge of the belly button.

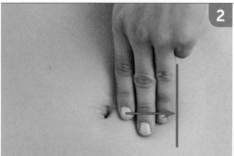

2 Where the third finger ends up on the abdomen, mark an imaginary vertical line. Slide the tip of the index finger along an imaginary horizontal line to the point where the two lines intersect. Where there is a slight depression you will find the point. Note the point.

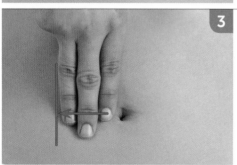

3 Next, locate the point on the opposite side of the abdomen.

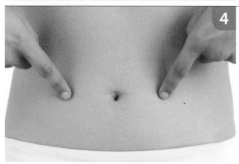

4 Using the index fingers, press both points at the same time.

Stomach 36

This point is located on the lower leg, one hand's width down from the knee crease, and one thumb's width lateral (to the right of) the shinbone.

Helps with these conditions

- bloating
- constipation and diarrhea
- all intestinal imbalances

- ulcer
- tinnitus (ringing in the ears)

- dizziness
- chills and fever
- grounding

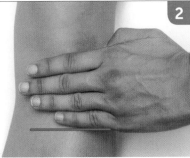
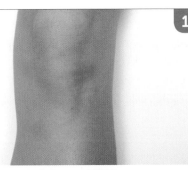
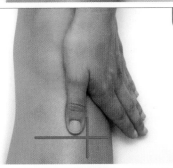
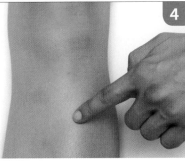

1 To locate the point, extend your leg while seated on a bed or floor.

2 Place your left hand on your right lower leg (shin) so that the index finger bumps up against the patella (kneecap). Where your pinky finger falls is the horizontal location line where you will find the point. Note the line and remove your left hand from your shin.

3 Next, place your right thumb vertically next to the shinbone so that the left edge of your thumb presses against the shinbone, and the widest part of your thumb falls across the horizontal line you just located. The right side of your thumb defines the vertical location line. Note this line.

4 Where these two location lines intersect is where you will find the point.

Stomach 40

This point is located on the lower leg.

Helps with these conditions

- phlegm
- cough
- wheezing
- pain and fullness in the chest and throat
- loss of voice
- bipolar disorder

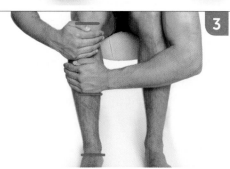

1 To locate the point, sit in a chair with both feet flat on the ground and the knees bent. Find the lower edge of the patella (kneecap). This is the upper location line. Note the line.

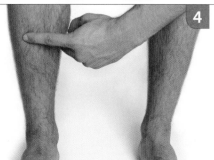

2 Next, locate the anterior (front) ankle crease. To find this line, with the index finger held horizontally, slide it from the toes up the foot until it runs into the ankle, right before the 90-degree bend created by the lower leg. This is the lower location line.

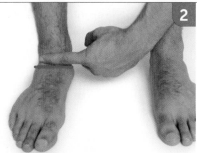

3 Next, slide the index finger down from the upper location line, along the tibia (shinbone) to find the midpoint between these two lines — it should be around two-hands width down from the upper location line.

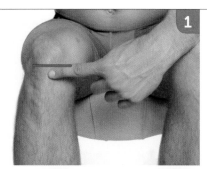

4 Slide the index finger laterally (to the outer side of the lower leg) along a horizontal line two fingers' width. This is where you will find the point.

Stomach 43

This point is located on the foot, between the second and third toes.

Helps with these conditions

- trigeminal neuralgia (facial nerve pain)
- edema
- swollen eyes
- abdominal fullness and gurgling

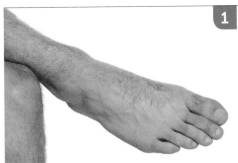

1 To locate the point, sit in a chair and cross one ankle over the opposite knee to allow easy access to the foot.

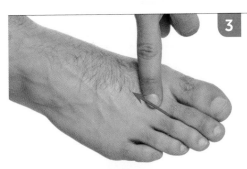

2 Find the toe crease between the second and third toes.

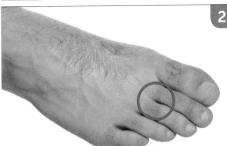

3 Slide the tip of the index finger from the toe crease up the foot, about two-fingers width above it.

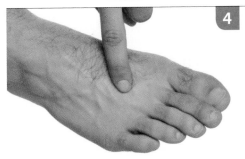

4 There are two distinct depressions. Where the finger lands on the second depression, furthest from the toes, is where you will find the point.

Spleen 4

This point is located on the medial (inner) side of the foot.

Helps with these conditions

- indigestion, especially with pain or cold sensation in the gastrointestinal tract (GI)
- bloating
- gurgling in the GI
- lack of appetite

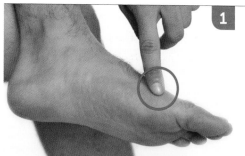

1 To locate the point, sit in a chair and cross one ankle over the opposite knee to allow easy access to the foot. Locate the large protruding bone at the first joint of the big toe.

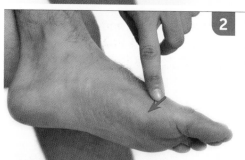

2 With an index finger, roll off the large bone diagonally, in the direction of the bottom of the foot until you feel the first long thin metatarsal bone.

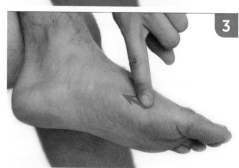

3 Next, slide the finger along the metatarsal bone toward the ankle. You should feel the large tendon on the bottom of the foot on the other side of your finger.

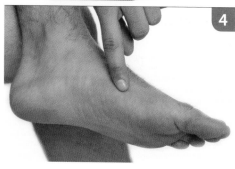

4 Continue to slide the index finger along the first metatarsal bone. Where it lands on a depression between the tendon of the foot and the upper end of the first metatarsal bone is where you will find the point.

Spleen 6

This point is located on the lower leg.

Warning: Avoid during pregnancy — can cause contractions.

Helps with these conditions

- allergies
- all female and male reproductive imbalances
- any digestive issues
- diabetes
- edema
- fungal infections
- nocturnal enuresis (bedwetting)

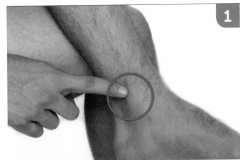

1 To locate the point, sit in a chair and cross one ankle over the opposite knee to allow easy access to the lower leg. Locate the medial malleolus (inner ankle bone).

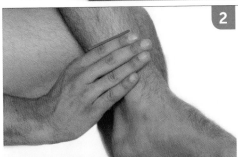

2 Next, place four fingers across the lower leg, with the outer edge of the fifth (pinky) finger pressing against the ankle bone. Note this line.

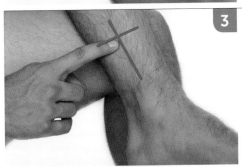

3 Locate the medial posterior (inner back) edge of the tibia (shinbone).

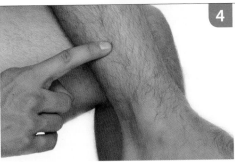

4 Where these two location lines intersect is where you will find the point.

Spleen 8

This point is located on the medial (inner) lower leg.

Helps with these conditions

- anemia
- irregular menstruation
- painful menstruation, especially acute onset

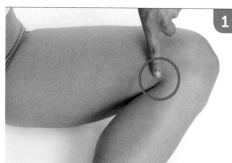

1 To locate the point, find the knee crease at the back of the leg, on the inner side.

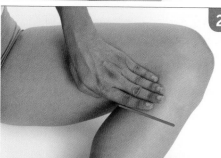

2 Place four fingers of one hand horizontally against the inner lower leg so that the fifth (pinky) finger lines up with the posterior (back) knee crease.

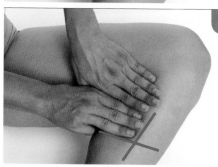

3 Next, place three fingers of the other hand immediately below the four fingers already on the lower leg so that seven fingers line up below the knee crease. Where the lower edge of the lowest finger intersects the back edge of the shinbone is where you will find the point.

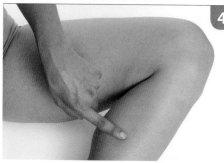

4 To find it, remove the first hand and palpate for the slight depression.

Spleen 10

This point is located on the medial (inner) leg just above the knee.

Helps with these conditions

- bruising and hematoma
- blood stasis
- blood deficiency
- excess bleeding
- varicosities (varicose veins, hemorrhoids)
- anemia in postpartum
- hot and itching conditions of the skin

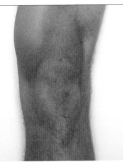

1 To locate the point, extend your legs while seated on a bed or floor.

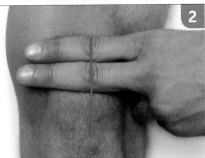

2 Place the index and middle fingers of one hand horizontally across the leg above the knee, so that the lower edge of the middle finger sits on the upper margin of the kneecap. The second joint of both fingers should be right above the center of the kneecap.

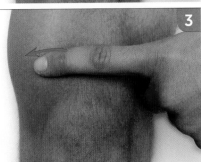

3 Next, slide the index finger medially (toward the inner thigh) about an inch (2.5 cm), so that the tip of the index finger lands about 1 inch further down the curve of the inner thigh than it was.

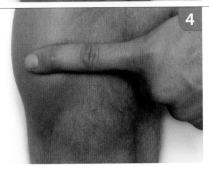

4 Where the tip of the index finger lands on a slight depression is where you will find the point.

Heart 7

This point is located on the forearm, at the wrist crease.

Helps with these conditions

- acute cold and flu symptoms, especially phlegm
- Raynaud syndrome
- headache due to stiff neck
- all postpartum imbalances
- depression

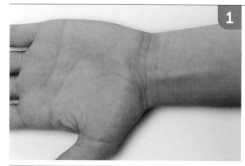

1 To locate the point, rest the hand on a comfortable surface, palm side facing up.

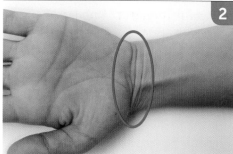

2 Locate the wrist crease by slightly bending the hand up. Relax the hand.

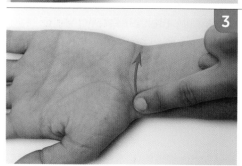

3 Next, slide the tip of the index finger along the wrist crease toward the pisiform (wrist) bone, the small bone of the wrist located directly beneath the fifth (pinky) finger.

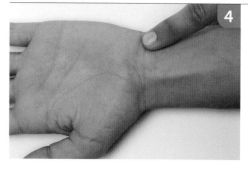

4 Where the wrist crease and the wrist bone meet is where you will find the point.

Small Intestine 1

This point is located on the fifth (pinky) finger, near the nail.

Helps with these conditions

- mastitis
- breast distention
- breast congestion
- clogged milk ducts

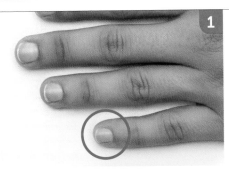

1 To locate the point, place the hand on a flat surface, palm side down. Find the bottom of the nail on the fifth (pinky) finger.

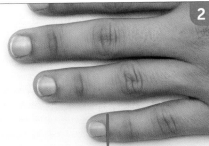

2 Note a location line at the bottom of the nail.

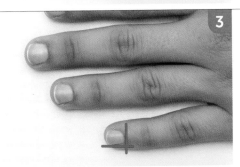

3 Next, note a line along the lateral (outer) side of the nail.

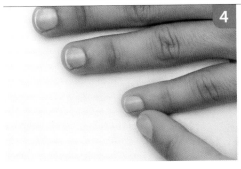

4 Where these two lines intersect is where you will find the point.

Small Intestine 3

This point is located on the lateral (outer) side of the hand.

Helps with these conditions

- arthritis
- torticollis (neck spasm, stiff neck)

- shaking or trembling limbs
- conditions related to the sensory organs

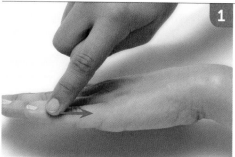

1 To locate the point, slide the tip of the index finger along the fifth (pinky) finger toward the wrist.

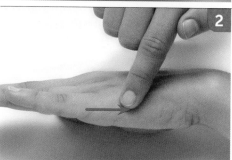

2 Slide the tip of the finger over the first joint of the pinky finger and onto a depression on the outer side of the hand.

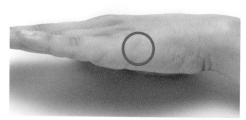

3 The depression lies between the hypothenar eminence (the pad on the outer edge of the palm) and the metacarpal of the pinky finger, the long bone along the side of the hand.

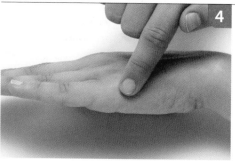

4 Where the finger lands on the center of this depression is where you will find the point.

Bladder 1

This point is located on the face, in between the nose and the inner corner of the eye (inner canthus), and slightly above it.

Helps with these conditions

- conjunctivitis (pinkeye) — treat the opposite eye
- excessive tearing

- most conditions of the eyes: dry, bloodshot, irritated, itching

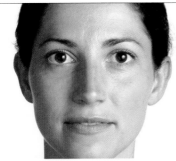

1 To locate the point, look at your face in a mirror.

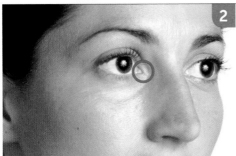

2 Locate the inner canthus, the area where the two eyelids come together, close to the nose.

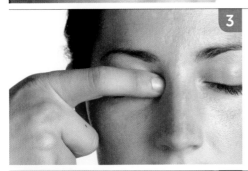

3 Next, gently place an index finger over the inner eyelid until the tip of the finger is resting in the inner canthus.

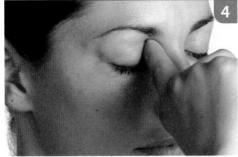

4 Very gently apply pressure to the eyeball while rolling the tip of the finger over it until the fingertip rolls over the innermost edge of the bone of the eye socket. Where the finger falls into the gap between the eyeball and the bone of the eye socket is where you will find the point. This point is held, not pressed.

Bladder 2

This point is located on the face, at the inner edge of the eyebrow.

Helps with these conditions

- allergies
- frontal headache
- blurred vision
- eyelid twitching
- rectal prolapse (protrusion)

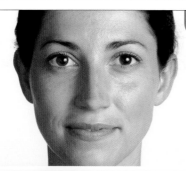

1 To locate the point, look at your face in a mirror.

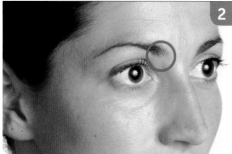

2 Locate the inner edge of the eyebrow.

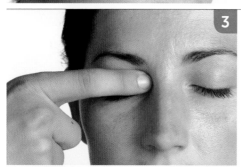

3 Next, locate the inner canthus of the eye, the area where the two eyelids come together, close to the nose.

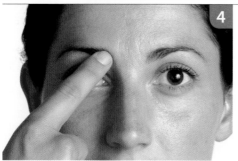

4 Slide the tip of the index finger from the hollow at the inner canthus up in the direction of the inner end of the eyebrow. Where the finger lands on a slight dip at the inner eyebrow is where you will find the point.

Bladder 9

This point is located on the back of the head, above the external occipital protuberance, the bony knob at the center of the back of the head.

Helps with these conditions

- occipital headache (headache at the back of the head)

- stiffness or heavy sensation of the neck

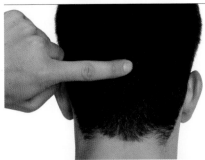

1 To locate the point, find the external occipital protuberance, the bump at the midline of the back of the head, approximately four fingers' width above the back hairline.

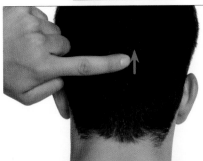

2 Roll an index finger over the bump to find a depression.

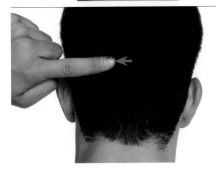

3 Continue to slide the finger up and out of the depression until it rests about an inch (2.5 cm) above it.

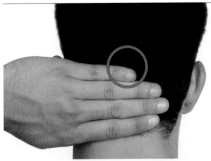

4 Next, slide the finger laterally about an inch. Where the finger lands on a slight depression, about one hand's width above the back hairline, is where you will find the point. This point is often tender to the touch. Locate the paired point on the other side in the same way, sliding laterally in the opposite direction.

Bladder 40

This point is located on the lower leg, on the back of the knee.

Helps with these conditions

- chronic or acute low back pain or stiffness
- chronic or acute knee pain or stiffness
- tendon stiffness
- all back pain

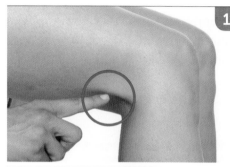

1 To locate the point, sit in a chair with both feet flat on the ground and the knees bent. Locate the tendon that defines the lateral (outside) border of the back of the knee.

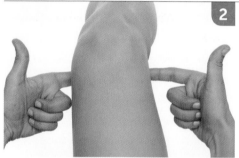

2 Next, locate the other tendons that define the medial (inner) border of the back of the knee. Both of these tendons can easily be felt when the knee is bent, by palpating with fingers behind the knee while tensing the muscles of the upper leg.

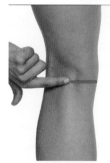
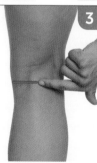

3 Next, with your index finger, reach into the soft tissue behind the knee at the level of the posterior knee crease.

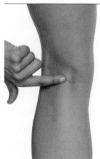
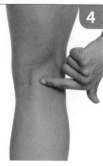

4 Where the finger lands on a depression at the center point midway between the two tendons is where you will find the point.

Bladder 67

This point is located on the outer edge of the fifth (pinky) toe.

Warning: Avoid during pregnancy — can cause contractions.

Helps with these conditions

- turning the fetus
- encouraging labor in pregnancy
- retained placenta
- heat in the head
- nasal congestion
- nosebleed
- heaviness in the head
- heat in the feet

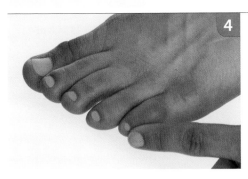

1 To locate the point, sit in a chair and cross one ankle over the opposite knee to allow easy access to the foot.

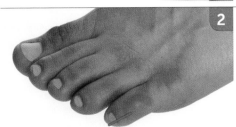

2 Locate the lateral (outer) edge of the toenail on the pinky toe and note this line.

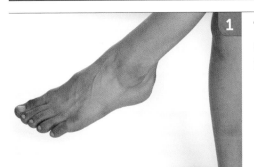

3 Next, locate the base of the toenail and note this line.

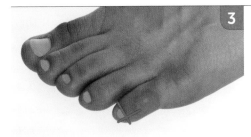

4 Where these two location lines intersect is where you will find the point.

Kidney 1

This point is located on the bottom of the foot.

Helps with these conditions

- plantar fasciitis
- anxiety
- insomnia

- lack of movement in the lower abdomen (constipation)

- dizziness
- difficulty urinating

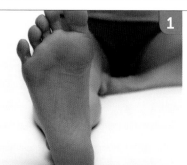

1 To locate the point, sit in a chair or on a flat surface.

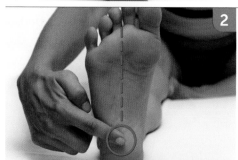

2 Locate the midline at the bottom of the foot.

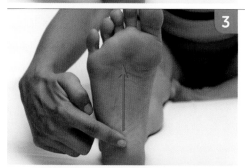

3 Next, slide your index finger along the midline of the sole of the foot toward the toes until it lands on the large depression just before the ball of the foot.

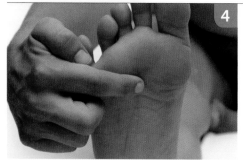

4 Where the finger lands on this depression is where you will find the point.

Kidney 3

This point is located on the medial (inner) ankle.

Helps with these conditions

- chronic/adrenal fatigue
- asthma
- seminal emissions
- excessive urination
- nocturnal enuresis (bedwetting, urinary incontinence)
- tinnitus (ringing in the ears)
- dizziness
- heat in the head
- cold at the extremities
- nosebleed and cough

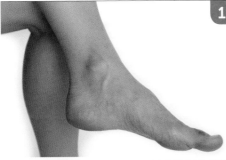

1 To locate the point, sit in a chair and cross one ankle over the opposite knee to allow easy access to the ankle.

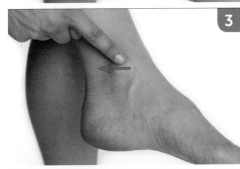

2 Locate the highest point of the medial malleolus (inner ankle bone).

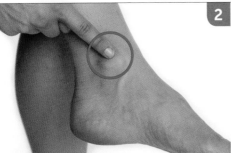

3 Next, from there, slide the tip of the index finger back toward the Achilles tendon, the large tendon that connects the calf to the foot, until the finger lands on a depression.

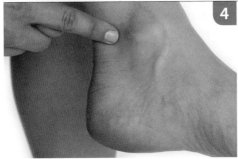

4 Where the finger lands on the center of this depression is where you will find the point.

Kidney 6

This point is located on the inner foot below the medial malleolus (inner ankle bone).

Helps with these conditions

- chronic fatigue
- hot flashes
- sore throat
- incontinence
- diarrhea
- menopausal symptoms
- leukorrhea (vaginal discharge)
- scanty menstruation

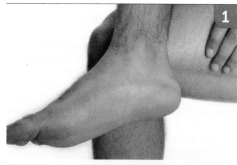

1 To locate the point, sit in a chair and cross one ankle over the opposite knee to allow easy access to the ankle.

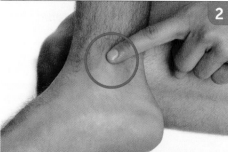

2 Locate your inner ankle bone.

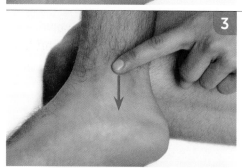

3 Next, from there, slide the tip of the index finger from the ankle bone down, until it drops into a depression located about one thumb's width below the bone.

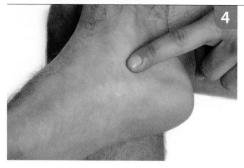

4 Where the finger lands on this depression is where you will find the point.

Kidney 7

This point is located on the inner part of the lower leg.

Helps with these conditions		
• edema (swelling), especially of the lower limbs	• dryness in the upper body, especially mouth, throat and nose	• spontaneous sweating • difficult urination • cystitis (bladder infections)

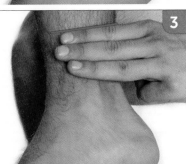

1 To locate the point, sit in a chair and cross one ankle over the opposite knee to allow easy access to the lower leg.

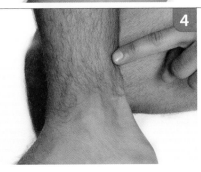

2 Locate the highest point of the medial malleolus (inner ankle bone).

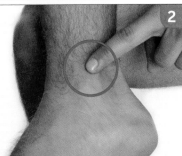

3 Measure three fingers' width up from the inner ankle bone to mark the upper horizontal location line. Note this line and remove your hand from that spot.

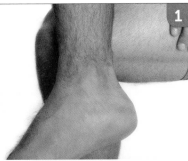

4 Next, on the same leg, find the Achilles tendon, the large tendon that runs up the back of the calf. Where the horizontal location line intersects with the inner edge of the Achilles tendon is where you will find the point.

Kidney 9

This point is located on the inner part of the lower leg.

Helps with these conditions

- feeling disconnected
- bipolar disorder
- anxiety
- insomnia
- lack of purpose
- heat in the upper body
- cold in the lower body

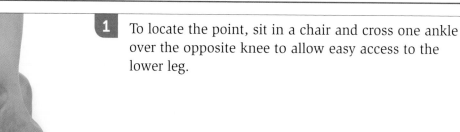

1 To locate the point, sit in a chair and cross one ankle over the opposite knee to allow easy access to the lower leg.

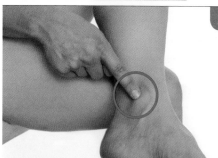

2 Locate the highest point of the medial malleolus (inner ankle bone).

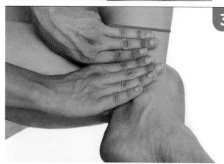

3 Next, measure seven fingers' width above the inner ankle bone. Note the horizontal line. The point is located one thumb's width from the inner edge of the tibia (shinbone) toward the calf.

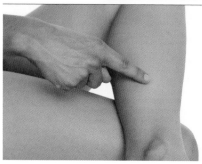

4 With the lower leg crossed and relaxed over the other leg, you will find the point approximately midway between the shin and the calf.

Kidney 26

This point is located on the upper chest, just under the second rib.

Helps with these conditions

- asthma, especially in adults
- phlegm
- palpitations
- drooling

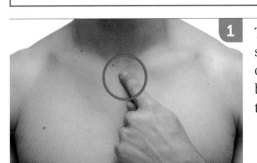 **1** To locate the point, use the index finger to find the sternum (breastbone), the large bone in the center of the chest where the ribs attach. At the top of the breastbone just below the throat, use the index finger to locate a notch.

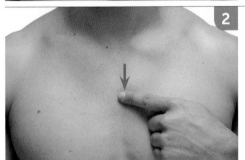 **2** From the notch, gently roll the index finger over the top of the sternum down toward the umbilicus (belly button) until it lands on a slight depression. This depression is aligned with the first intercostal space; that is, the gap beneath the first rib.

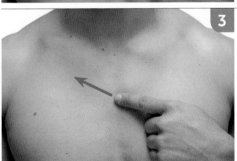 **3** Next, slide the tip of the finger laterally (away from the sternum) up and over the connection between the first rib and the sternum, approximately three fingers' width from the center of the sternum until it lands on a depression.

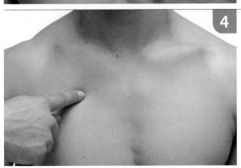 **4** Roll the tip of the finger down, over the second rib, until it is in the corresponding depression in the second intercostal space. Where the tip of the finger falls on the center of this depression is where you will find the point.

Kidney 27

This point is located on the upper chest, just under the clavicle.

Helps with these conditions

- asthma especially in children
- chronic cough

- phlegm, nausea and vomiting, especially vomiting phlegm

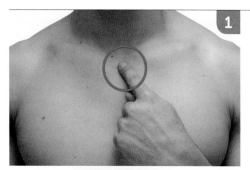

1 To locate the point, use the index finger to find the sternum (breastbone), the large bone in the center of the chest where the ribs attach.

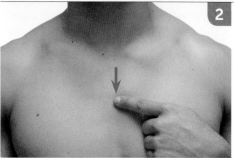

2 At the top of the breastbone just below the throat, use the index finger to locate a notch. From the notch, gently roll the finger over the top of the sternum until it lands on a depression. This depression is aligned with the first intercostal space; that is, the gap beneath the first rib.

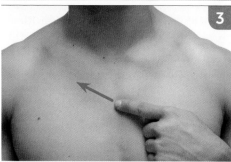

3 Next, slide the tip of the finger laterally (away from the sternum) up and over the connection between the first rib and the sternum, approximately three fingers' width from the center of the sternum until it lands on a depression.

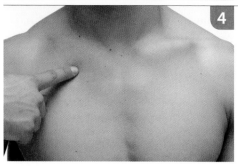

4 Where the tip of the finger lands on the center of this depression is where you will find the point.

Pericardium 6

This point is located on the medial (inner) forearm close to the wrist.

Helps with these conditions

- addiction
- angina pectoris (chest pain)

- nausea and vomiting
- morning sickness
- anxiety

- insomnia
- conditions of the chest

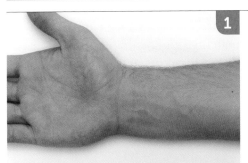

1 To locate the point, rest the arm on a comfortable surface, palm side facing up.

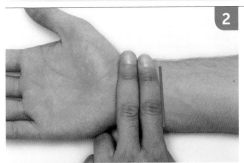

2 Place two middle fingers from your left hand on your right forearm so that the middle finger lays facedown over the wrist crease. Where the index finger falls is the horizontal location line. Note the line and remove your left hand from your forearm.

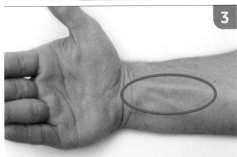

3 Next, locate the tendon in the center of the forearm by bending your hand at the wrist so that the palm is moving up, toward the elbow.

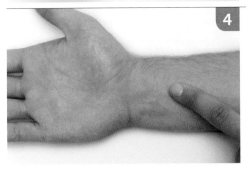

4 Where the horizontal location line intersects the tendon is where you will find the point. Bring your hand back down before pressing the point.

Pericardium 7

This point is located on the medial (inner) forearm, on the wrist crease.

Helps with these conditions

- carpal tunnel syndrome
- heart pain
- palpitations
- shortness of breath
- fullness or pain in the chest

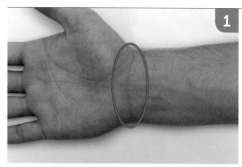

1 To locate the point, rest the hand on a comfortable surface, palm side facing up. Locate the wrist crease by slightly bending the hand up. Relax the hand.

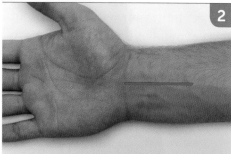

2 Next, locate the tendon at the center of the wrist.

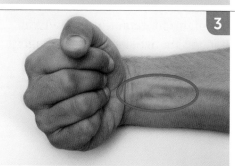

3 Tensing all fingers will engage the tendon, making it easier to find.

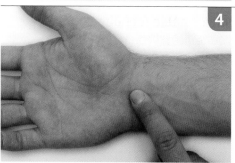

4 Where the wrist crease and the tendon intersect is where you will find the point.

Triple Warmer 3

This point is located on the dorsal (back) side of the hand.

Helps with these conditions

- tinnitis (ringing in the ears), especially sudden onset
- earache, especially due to exposure to cold wind
- deafness
- one-sided headache

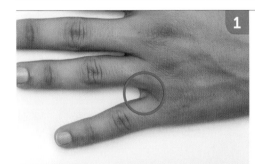

1 To locate the point, find the webbing between the fourth (ring) and fifth (pinky) fingers.

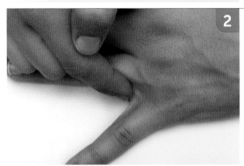

2 With the opposite hand, slide the tip of the index finger from the webbing between the fourth and fifth finger toward the wrist, sliding just over the bones of the first joint between the fingers and the hand and into the first depression.

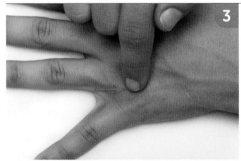

3 The finger's tip should be about two fingers' width from the end of the webbing between the two fingers.

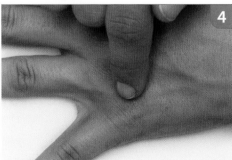

4 Where the finger lands on this first depression is where you will find the point.

Triple Warmer 14

This point is located on the posterior (back) shoulder, at the shoulder joint.

Helps with these conditions

- adhesive capsulitis (frozen shoulder), especially at the back of the shoulder
- numbness or pain of the shoulder or arm

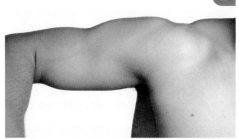

1 To locate the point, stand in front of a mirror. Bend the arm 90 degrees and raise the elbow until it is level with the shoulder.

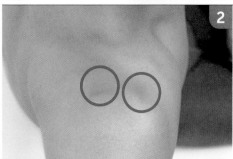

2 This will cause two depressions to appear next to each other at the top of the shoulder. If they are not obvious, palpate for them just above the deltoid muscle at the top of the arm.

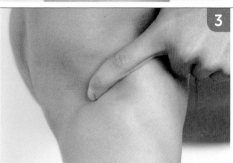

3 Next, use the index finger from the opposite hand to find the posterior depression (in the back).

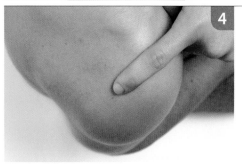

4 Where the finger lands on the depression closest to the back is where you will find the point. Be sure to relax the arm before pressing the point.

Triple Warmer 21

This point is located on the face, just in front of the ear.

Helps with these conditions

- trigeminal neuralgia (facial nerve pain)
- deafness
- tinnitus (ringing in the ears)
- ear infection
- toothache

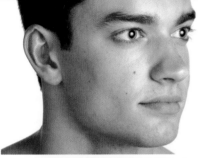

1 To locate the point, stand in front of a mirror.

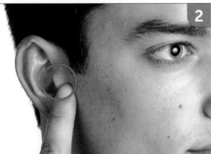

2 Locate the tragus, the small flap of cartilage at the front of the ear. This is the part we sometimes press on to block sound.

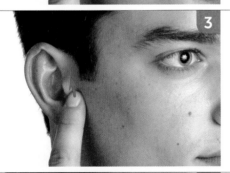

3 Next, at the point where the ear attaches to the head close to the front hairline, roll the tip of the index finger up the edge of the face, to the depression just above the tragus (flap).

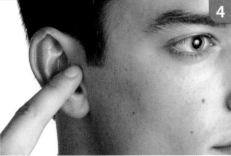

4 Where the finger lands on the center of this depression is where you will find the point.

Gallbladder 3

This point is located on either side of the face.

Helps with these conditions

- tinnitus (ringing in the ears)
- ear conditions of all types
- gum disease
- toothache of the upper jaw
- temporomandibular joint (TMJ) pain

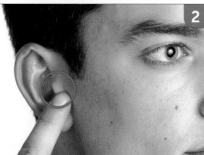

1 To locate the point, stand in front of a mirror.

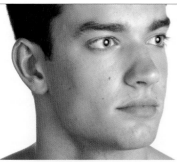

2 Locate the tragus, the small flap of cartilage at the front of the ear. This is the part we sometimes press on to block sound.

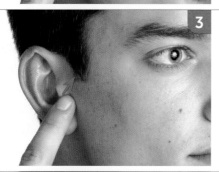

3 Next, slide the finger along the cheekbone and away from the ear in the direction of the nose to locate the bottom edge of the zygomatic arch (cheekbone), about one thumbs' width from the starting point, until the tip of the finger lands on a depression.

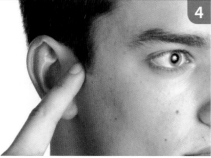

4 Where the finger finds the center of this depression is where you will find the point.

Gallbladder 6

This point is located on the side of the head, above and slightly forward of the ear, on the temple.

Helps with these conditions

- one-sided headache
- temporal headache
- fever headache

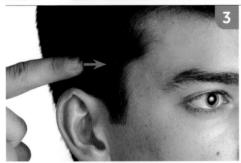

1 To locate the point, stand in front of a mirror.

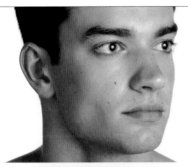

2 Slide the tip of the index finger up from the top of the ear to just about one finger's width above it.

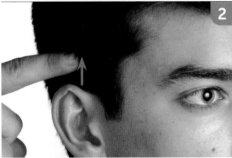

3 Next, slide the finger directly forward toward the eyebrow, about one finger's width until the tip of the finger lands on a depression.

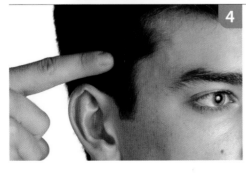

4 Where the finger lands on the center of this depression is where you will find the point.

Gallbladder 14

This point is located on the forehead.

Helps with these conditions

- frontal headache
- eye pain
- pain on the face
- eyelid twitching
- eyelid droop, especially post stroke

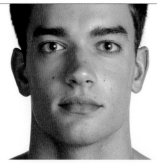

1 To locate the point, stand in front of a mirror.

2 Locate the vertical pupil line in the eye; that is, the vertical line that runs through the center of the pupil. This often cuts through the center of the highest part of the eyebrow.

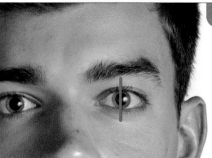

3 Next, slide the tip of the index finger about one finger's width above the eyebrow.

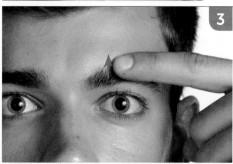

4 Where the finger lands on the center of the slight depression is where you will find this point.

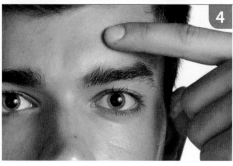

Gallbladder 20

This point is located on the back of the head.

Helps with these conditions

- insomnia
- all conditions on the face
- temporal headache
- one-sided headache
- stiffness and rigidity of the neck
- lacrimation (excessive tearing, especially due to wind)

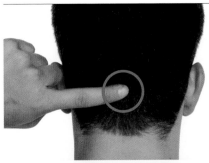

1 To locate the point, find the external occipital protuberance, the bony prominence at the back of the head, about one hand's width above the back hairline.

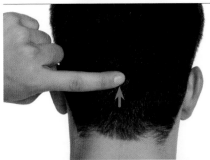

2 Slide the tip of the index finger over this prominence until it lands on a depression.

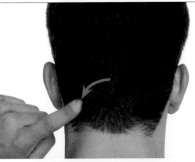

3 Next, move the index finger laterally (to the outer side) along the bony ridge about three fingers' width, until it hits a fleshy mound.

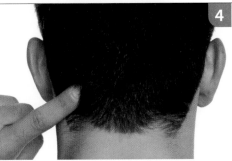

4 Where the finger lands in the center of this mound is where you will find the point.

Gallbladder 30

This point is located on the buttocks.

Helps with these conditions

- sciatica
- pain in the hip or buttock
- lumbar pain
- pain or numbness in the leg
- atrophy of the limbs

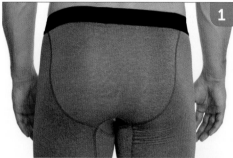

1 To locate the point, stand in a relaxed position.

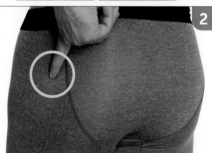

2 With your fingers, find the large depression at the center of one of the buttock cheeks.

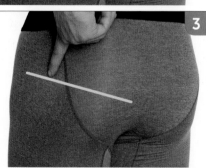

3 This point falls on a line drawn from the tip of the coccyx (tailbone) to the hip socket.

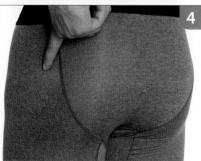

4 Where the finger lands on the center of this depression is where you will find the point.

Gallbladder 34

This point is located on the lower leg, near the knee.

Helps with these conditions

- disorders of the sinews, tendons, ligaments and connective tissue
- most nerve disorders
- stiffness in the limbs (especially knees)
- atrophy of the limbs
- trigeminal neuralgia (facial nerve pain); sciatica

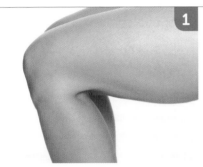

1 To locate the point, sit in a chair with both feet flat on the ground and the knees bent.

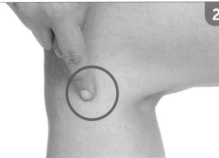

2 With your fingers, locate the fibula bone, found toward the outside of the leg, next to the larger tibia (shinbone).

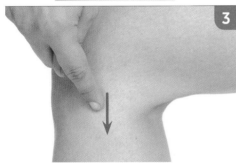

3 Next, slide the finger down from the knee until it lands on a large depression just under the head of the fibula. The head of the fibula articulates with the knee, so the location of this point is quite close to the knee.

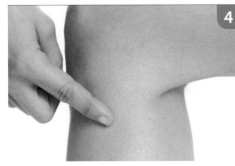

4 Where your finger lands, about three fingers' width below the level of the posterior (back) knee crease, is where you will find the point.

Gallbladder 43

This point is located on the foot.

Helps with these conditions

- throbbing in the head upon standing
- hypertension
- red eyes
- fullness of the chest

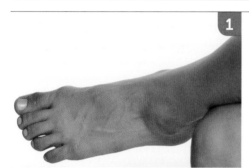

1 To locate the point, sit in a chair and cross the ankle over the opposite knee to allow easy access to the foot.

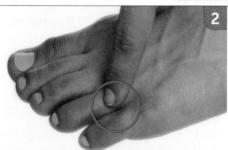

2 Locate the toe crease between the fourth and fifth toes.

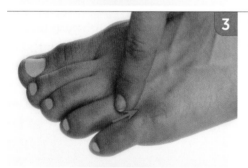

3 Next, slide your finger in the direction of the ankle along the toe crease.

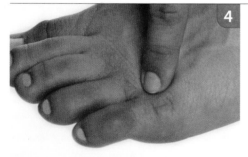

4 Where the tip of the finger slides up just barely out of the toe crease is where you will find the point.

Liver 2

This point is located on the top of the foot.

Helps with these conditions

- prostatitis and prostate infections
- heat and pain in the head and throat
- cold limbs
- tendency toward anger

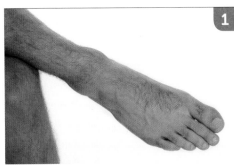

1 To locate the point, sit in a chair and cross one ankle over the opposite knee to allow easy access to the foot.

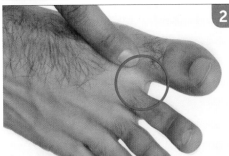

2 Locate the webbing between the big and second toes.

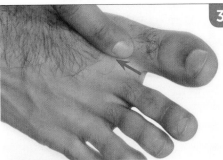

3 Next, slide the tip of the index finger along the valley between the tendons of these two toes in the direction of the ankle. Make sure the tip of the finger is centered between the tendons of the big toe and the second toe.

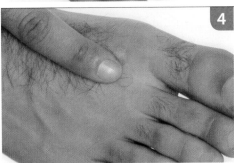

4 Continue sliding the finger — where it lands on a slight depression, about one-half a thumb's width from the end of the toe crease, is where you will find the point.

Liver 3

This point is located on the top of the foot.

Helps with these conditions

- hepatitis
- spasmodic cough
- abdominal pain

- genital pain
- difficulty arising upon waking

- dizziness
- shortness of breath
- irregular menstruation

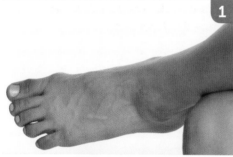

1 To locate the point, sit in a chair and cross one ankle over the opposite knee to allow easy access to the foot.

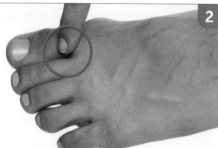

2 Locate the webbing between the big and second toes.

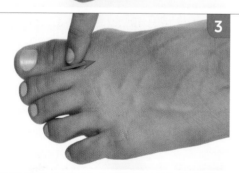

3 Next, slide the tip of the index finger along the valley between the tendons of these two toes until it lands on a depression, about one thumb's width from the end of the toe crease. Make sure the tip of the finger is centered between the tendons of the big toe and the second toe.

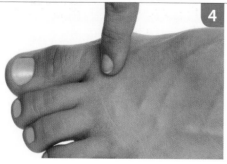

4 Where the finger lands on the center of this depression is where you will find the point.

Liver 8

This point is located on the leg, close to the medial (inner) knee.

Helps with these conditions

- anxiety manifesting as mania
- impotence
- itching of the genitals
- leukorrhea (vaginal discharge)
- spermatorrhea (involuntary ejaculation)

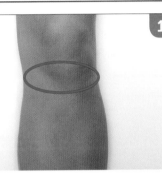

1 To locate the point, extend the leg and find the bottom edge of the patella (kneecap).

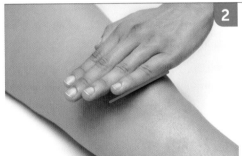

2 Lay four fingers across the kneecap on the opposite leg so that the outer edge of the fifth (pinky) finger sits at the bottom of the kneecap. The index finger should be resting on a line that extends through the fleshy tissue on the inner leg.

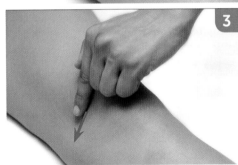

3 Next, slide the tip of the index finger about an inch down the curve of the inner thigh until it is on the highest point of this fleshy area.

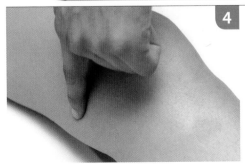

4 Where the tip of the finger rests on this highest point is where you will find the point.

Conception Vessel 1

This point is located on the perineum, the small space between the external genitals and the anus.

Helps with these conditions

- all conditions of the reproductive organs and anus
- bowel incontinence
- prostatitis (prostate infection)
- shock
- history of fainting spells
- vaginal candida

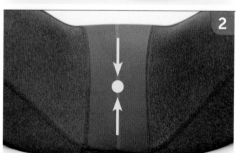

1 To locate the point, find the perineum between the genitals and anus.

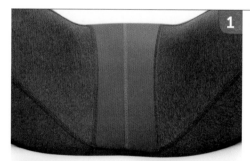

2 Slide the index finger to find the spot midway between these two reference points.

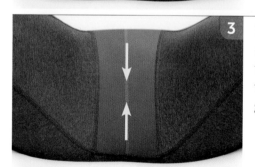

3 If the tip of the index finger slides too far up to the external genitalia, it needs to move further down toward the anus. If the finger slides too far toward the anus, it needs to move back toward the external genitalia, until it is directly between the two.

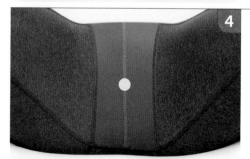

4 The center point between these reference points is where you will find the point.

Conception Vessel 3

This point is located on the lower abdomen.

Warning: Avoid during pregnancy — may cause too much pressure on the baby.

Helps with these conditions

- incontinence
- pain below the umbilicus (belly button)
- low back pain
- excess or deficient menstruation
- uterine prolapse
- retention of placenta in childbirth

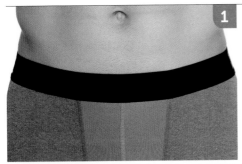

1 To locate the point, stand in front of a mirror. Expose the lower abdomen.

2 Locate the superior border of the pubic symphysis, the bone usually found just above the public hair, about eight fingers' width directly below the umbilicus (belly button). Place an index finger on it.

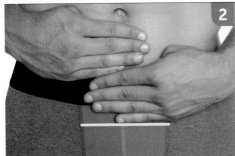

3 Next, slide the tip of the finger up one thumb's width toward the belly button until it lands on a slight depression.

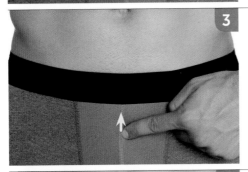

4 Where the tip of the finger lands on the center of this depression is where you will find the point.

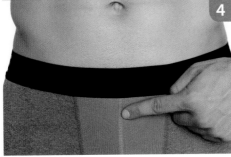

Conception Vessel 4

This point is located on the lower abdomen.

Warning: Avoid during pregnancy — may cause too much pressure on the baby.

Helps with these conditions

- exhaustion
- weakness
- low-back pain

- deficiency conditions of all kinds

- infertility
- urinary incontinence

- muscle atrophy (shrinking/wasting of the limbs)

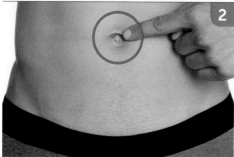

1 To locate the point, stand in front of a mirror. Expose the lower abdomen.

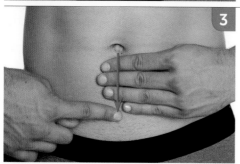

2 Locate the umbilicus (belly button). Place a finger on it.

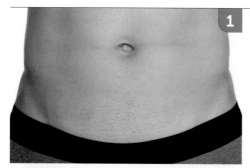

3 Next, slide the finger down about four fingers' width.

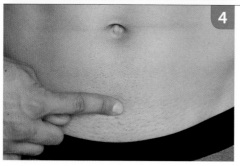

4 Where the finger lands on the swell of tissue just under the belly button is where you will find the point.

Conception Vessel 10

This point is located on the abdomen.

Warning: Avoid during pregnancy — may cause too much pressure on the baby.

Helps with these conditions

- indigestion
- food stagnation
- undigested food in the stool
- nausea or vomiting, especially after eating

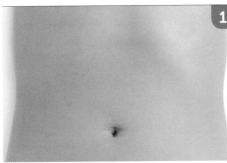

1 To locate the point, stand in front of a mirror. Expose the abdomen.

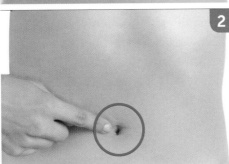

2 Locate the umbilicus (belly button). Place a finger on it.

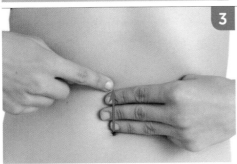

3 Next, slide the tip of the index finger three fingers' width up from the umbilicus (belly button).

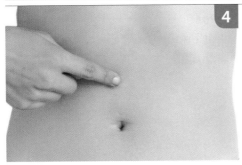

4 Where the finger lands on a depression is where you will find the point.

Conception Vessel 12

This point is located on the abdomen.
Warning: Avoid during pregnancy — may cause too much pressure on the baby.

Helps with these conditions

- all digestive conditions
- diarrhea
- GERD (heartburn, acid reflux)
- lack of appetite
- the habit of eating to relieve stress
- easily feeling full
- vomiting

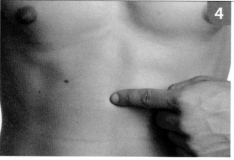

1 To locate the point, stand in front of a mirror. Expose the abdomen.

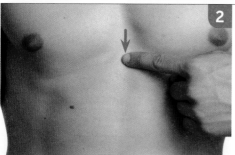

2 Slide the index finger to locate the bottom of the xiphoid process, the lower end of the sternum (breastbone). If the xiphoid itself cannot be located, find the point where the ribs join the low end of the sternum as a reference point.

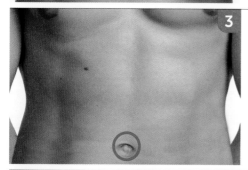

3 Next, locate the umbilicus (belly button).

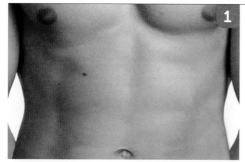

4 The midway point between these two structures, about six fingers' width down from the sternum or up from the belly button, is where you will find the point.

Conception Vessel 17

This point is located on the chest, directly over the sternum (breastbone).

Helps with these conditions

- any conditions of the chest
- asthma
- shortness of breath
- pain with breathing
- acid reflux
- esophageal constriction
- insufficient lactation during breastfeeding

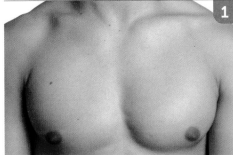

1 To locate the point, stand in front of a mirror. Expose the chest.

2 Slide the index finger along the rib cage to locate the fourth intercostal space, the space just below the fourth rib. This can be felt more easily by palpating the area off of the sternum, as shown. This space is about five fingers' width below where the clavicle (collarbone) meets the sternum (breastbone).

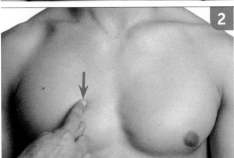

3 From the rib, slide the tip of the index finger medially (toward the center) until the finger rests on the sternum at the point level with the fourth intercostal space.

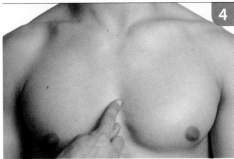

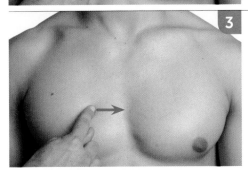

4 This is where you will find the point. For women, this point may be more easily found while lying down in order to move breast tissue out of the way.

Conception Vessel 22

This point is located on the lower neck.

Helps with these conditions

- cough with thin, colorless secretions
- esophageal constriction
- persistent tickle in the throat
- loss of voice
- dry throat
- thyroid imbalance

1 To locate the point, stand in front of a mirror.

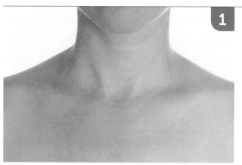

2 Slide the index finger over the sternum (breastbone) to find the notch in the center of the top of this bone.

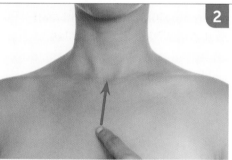

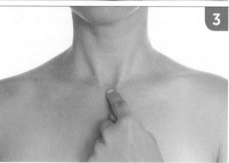

3 The point is actually located behind the bone, so it is best pressed by gently rolling the finger up and over the breastbone, into the hollow behind it.

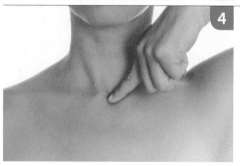

4 Be careful not to apply pressure to the hyoid bone (Adam's apple), which is located just above this point.

Conception Vessel 23

This point is located on the upper neck, just under the chin.

Helps with these conditions

- aphthous ulcers (mouth sores)
- halitosis (bad breath)
- bleeding gums
- excessive or deficient salivation
- vomiting foam

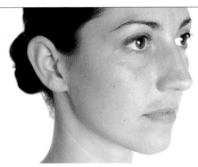

1 To locate the point, stand in front of a mirror.

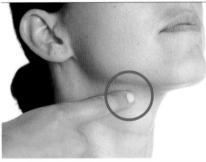

2 Locate the juncture where the neck and the chin come together at midline (center of the neck).

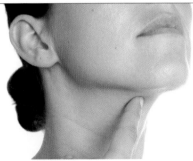

3 It is easiest to locate this point when the head is at a neutral position, facing forward, chin slightly raised. When the point is pressed, it will be felt at the root (back) of the tongue.

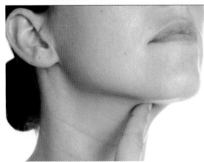

4 Next, press the point gently with the index finger approximately at a 45-degree angle, in order to avoid closing the trachea (airways). Avoid putting pressure on the hyoid bone (Adam's apple), which is located just below this point.

Governing Vessel 20

This point is located on the top of the head.

Helps with these conditions

- vertex headache (pain at the top of the head)
- dizziness upon standing
- vertigo and light-headedness
- uterine or rectal prolapse
- poor memory
- foggy brain

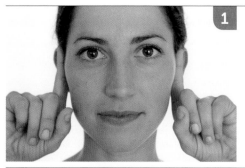

1 To locate the point, stand in front of a mirror. Place both index fingers along the side of the face where the ear attaches to the face.

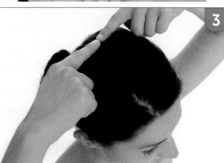

2 Next, follow an imaginary line that runs from the front of each ear to the top of the head.

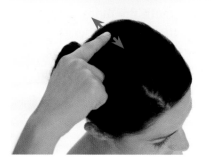

3 Where these two lines intersect at the top of the head, approximately eight fingers' width from the anterior (front) hairline, is where you will find the point.

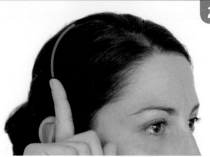

4 For some people, this point may be slightly anterior (forward) or posterior (behind) — it is usually tender or sensitive, so it is easily located by a sensation of tenderness.

Governing Vessel 26

This point is located on the face.

Helps with these conditions

- sudden loss of consciousness
- bipolar disorder
- nosebleed
- runny nose

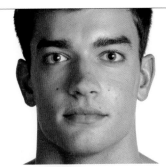

1 To locate the point, stand in front of a mirror.

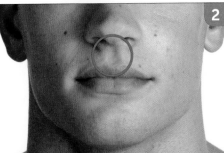

2 Locate the philtrum, the space beneath the nose, between the two nostrils and the upper lip.

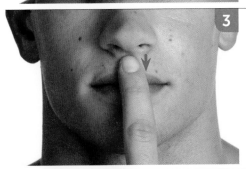

3 Next, with a fingernail pressing against the bottom of the center of the nose, slide the tip of the finger slightly down toward the mouth.

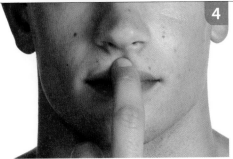

4 Where the tip of the fingernail is resting on a slight depression in the center of the philtrum, just above the upper lip, is where you will find the point. The curve of the upper gum can be felt beneath the pad of the finger, through the lip.

Dingchuan

This point is located on the back of the neck.

Helps with these conditions

- asthma
- cough
- wheezing
- shortness of breath

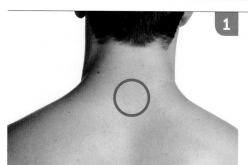

1 To locate the point, find the large spinous process of the first thoracic (T1) vertebra, which is the large knob at the very top of the spine.

2 To ensure you are on the correct vertebra, with the index finger on the large knob, rotate your head left and then right, as though you are looking over your shoulder. The vertebra should not move. If it does, slide your finger down to the first vertebra that does not move.

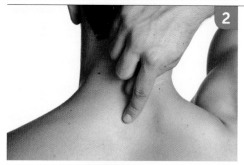

3 Next, slip the tip of the index finger into the depression just above the large knob.

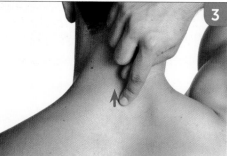

4 Slide the tip of the finger laterally (away from the spine) one finger's width until it lands on a depression. With the tip of your other finger, slide laterally in the other direction to find the paired point. Where the fingers land on these depressions is where you will find the points.

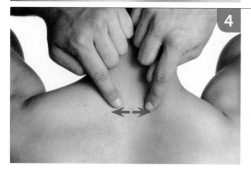

Yintang

This point is located on the face, between the eyebrows.

Helps with these conditions

- fright
- insomnia
- restlessness
- agitation

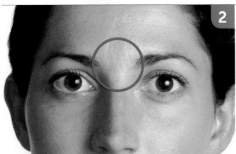

1 To locate the point, stand in front of a mirror.

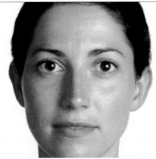

2 Locate the area between the eyebrows. There may be a raised area or it may be flat.

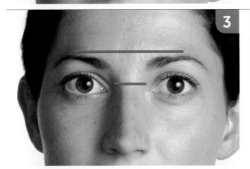

3 Next, find the horizontal location line that marks the highest point of the brows. Note this line. Find the groove that marks the bottom of the square between the brows. Note this groove.

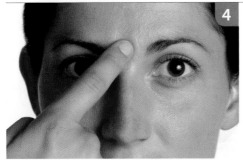

4 At the very center of the square defined by the horizontal location line and the groove is where you will find the point. For many people, the point is equidistant from the inner ends of the eyebrows and the groove that marks the bottom of the square between the brows.

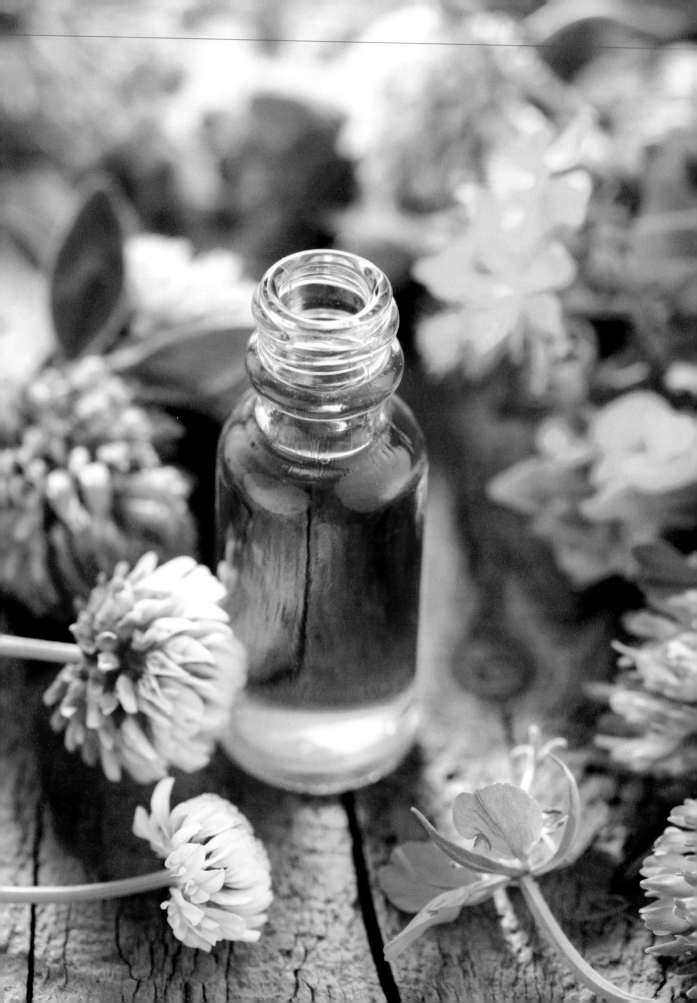

CHAPTER 3

Aromatherapy: Using Essential Oils for Health Conditions

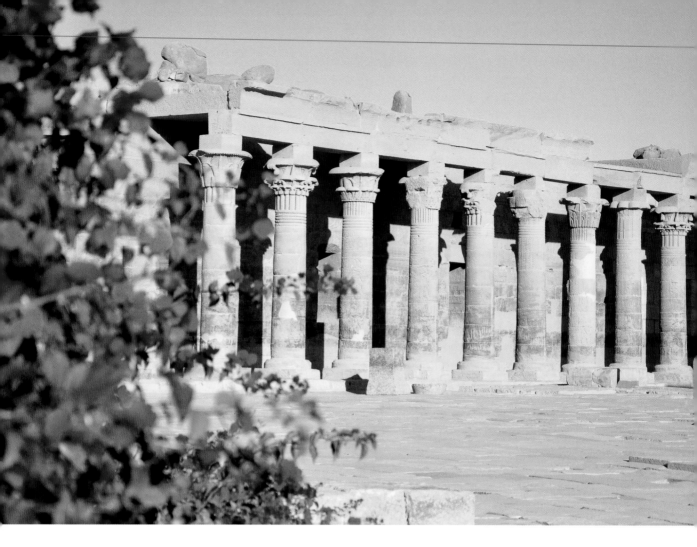

History of Fragrance

Humans have used fragrance, either natural or synthetic, throughout history. Thousands of years ago, most of the exposure to "perfumes" was probably a side effect of using plants for healing, but I like to imagine ancient civilizations delighting in beautiful scents as an experience in itself. Centuries later, fragrances were being manufactured to use as scents (although some would argue this was just to cover the stink of humanity, I admit to being a romantic and choose to see it differently).

In some cases, there was no distinction between medicines and scenting agents. A good example is a substance used by the ancient Egyptians called kyphi, which has been documented as a substance used both for medicinal and ceremonial purposes. The Egyptians also used an interesting delivery mechanism called the bitcone. These cones were made of fats embedded with fragrant plant material, often from the same plants used to make incense (such as kyphi). The cones were placed on a person's head and eventually melted over the body. They can often be seen in hieroglyphs at burial sites, indicating they were quite common.

The use of incense in Asia can be traced back thousands of years. There is evidence that incense was being used in ancient China as early as 2000 BCE. Japan, known in modern times for producing the finest incenses available, was introduced to the art by monks traveling from Korea. As with many practices, Japanese practitioners have elevated the use of incense to an art form and still perform incense ceremonies.

Extracting Essential Oils

Essential oils (EOs) differ from the plant-based creations discussed earlier because the whole plant is not used in extractions. Each oil is created from different parts of the plant — rose petals are used for rose essential oil, for example, or fennel seeds for fennel essential oil. Some plants offer up different oils from each of their various plant parts. For example, sweet orange essential oil is made from the rind of the fruit, neroli essential oil is derived from orange blossoms, and the green twigs and leaves of the bitter orange produce petitgrain essential oil.

The essence of the plant is captured through various means, but primarily through a process known as distillation. Distillation appears to have arisen in many parts of the world at around the same time. The Greek alchemists in Alexandria worked extensively with the process of evaporation and condensation, and passed the tools of this process on to the Arab world, where the technique was preserved.

Methods of Extraction

Steam Distillation

To this day, steam distillation is the most common means of extracting essential oils from plants. Here is how the process works: the plant material is loaded into the top section of a distillation device. The bottom is filled with water that is then heated to produce steam. As the pressure builds, the steam is forced through the plant matter, which liberates the essential oils. The mixture of water and oil is then passed through a coil immersed in cold water, which forces the two to separate. From the coil, it passes into a receiving vat. The final step is removing the lighter essential oils floating on the surface of the water. The water that remains is also used in aromatherapy. It goes by several different names but is most commonly called hydrosol.

Expression

Expression is the technique used for plants that store their essential oils in the skin of the fruits they produce. These are mostly the citrus oils, such as lemon and grapefruit. It is quite easy to access these essential oils — if you have ever peeled an orange and seen the fine mist spraying from the peel (which seems to always, inevitably, end up in someone's eye), you have expressed an essential oil. For mass production, a large press is used.

Enfleurage

Enfleurage is an old technique that has mostly been abandoned, except by the most dedicated natural perfumers, since it is a long and labor-intensive process designed to remove scent molecules from delicate flower petals that cannot withstand steam distillation. During this process, a layer of solid fat is painted onto a smooth, flat surface, such as marble or glass. Flower petals are meticulously laid down on the fat and left for a day or two. When all the scent has been removed, the spent flowers are stripped off and a new layer is added. This procedure may be repeated dozens of times before the fat is washed with alcohol to separate the essential oils. After the alcohol is allowed to evaporate, the remaining substance is called an absolute.

Chemical Extraction

Nowadays, most absolutes are created by chemical extraction. Hexane is commonly used as a solvent and, despite being quite volatile, never completely leaves the absolute. It is nearly impossible to find organically certified absolutes, but because the substances left behind in this process are mostly used in perfumery and not for medical aromatherapy, it is not an issue for our purposes.

In recent years, a newer method — carbon dioxide (CO_2) extraction — has offered exciting possibilities. When gaseous CO_2 is put under enough pressure, it becomes a liquid that is particularly good at liberating essential oils. An added bonus is that many compounds poorly extracted by water (steam distillation) — substances like waxy fatty acids, for example — are easily accessed by CO_2 extraction. This adds depth and richness to the resulting oils. The best part, however, is that when the process is finished, the pressure is released and the CO_2 returns to its gas form, leaving behind a pure essential oil with no residues.

Sourcing Essential Oils

Always look for the purest essential oils processed from organic plant matter when using them for medical aromatherapy. This is the only way to ensure we are promoting good health with these medicinal substances.

Systems and Order

To be clinically useful, any system of medicine must have order. Cultures around the world have interacted with plants for millennia, so it is not surprising that many different systems have developed. Many people first learn about essential oils from a symptom-based perspective; that is, the experience of a symptom is an opportunity to learn about the oils that can treat it. Many books on essential oils offer lists of oils categorized in this way. There is an element of rote learning to this system, as no overarching concept is applied — it is more of a piecemeal approach. It relies on observations made in the home or possibly the clinical setting.

Many indications have been passed down traditionally from teachers or colleagues. These observations carry a lot of historical weight but, again, do not conform to a theoretical or philosophical model, for the most part.

Medical Aromatherapy

Also called modern aromatherapy, medical aromatherapy is a fairly recent development. The rise of this practice is credited to French chemist René-Maurice Gattefossé, considered the founder of modern medical aromatherapy. A well-known story in the world of aromatherapy comes from Gattefossé's 1937 book, *Aromathérapie* (translated into English in 1977 by Robert Tisserand), in which he talks about how the application of lavender oil dramatically reduced healing time for a burn he sustained in the lab:

> *The external application of small quantities of essences rapidly stops the spread of gangrenous sores. In my personal experience, after a laboratory explosion covered me with burning substances which I extinguished by rolling on a grassy lawn, both my hands were covered with a rapidly developing gas gangrene. Just one rinse with lavender essence stopped the "gasification of the tissue." This treatment was followed by profuse sweating, and healing began the next day (July 1910).*

The remarkable results lead Gattefossé to devote his attention to the study of essential oils and we can say that modern aromatherapy was born.

Modern Aromatherapy as Medicine

Unlike the traditional approach, modern Western (or medical) aromatherapy does have a theoretical model. The system is based on the primary chemical constituents found in each oil; for example, an oil may be classified as a monoterpene or an aldehyde because that is the chemical constituent that makes up the bulk of the oil (in some cases, the action of a constituent that makes up a small percentage of the oil is nevertheless the strongest). Rather than selecting an oil based on traditional indications, the oil is chosen because its major constituent is known to have a beneficial effect to treat the condition. For example, α-santalol, found in sandalwood essential oil, has been shown to be effective against the bacteria that cause urinary tract infections. When addressing this condition, sandalwood oil is used because it contains α-santalol and not because it has traditionally been used in this way. (For more information on the properties of essential oils, see chart page 109.)

The prevalence of the constituent-based system in medical aromatherapy makes sense — modern pharmaceutical medicine works in a very similar way and it is considered the standard of care. The prevailing biochemical approach of modern medicine is excellent for understanding the gross effects of the undiluted chemical constituent, for example, but less able to measure the subtle effects occurring on the bioenergetic — how energy transforms in living organisms. While aromatherapy that is appropriately delivered can frequently effect change in the bioenergetic milieu, the modern approach still misses a lot.

Measuring Bioenergetic Benefits

Understanding all of the minute shifts occurring in cellular metabolism, for example, requires a dramatic readjustment of focus, down to the very smallest level of activity. Many subtle changes are happening that are difficult to observe and even more difficult to measure.

Most natural medicine systems are not tested or understood within the system from which they arose. Instead, practitioners, researchers and educators are expected to work within the language and ideas of the prevailing paradigm of conventional medicine. This language has always been difficult to navigate for many reasons.

First, nature is infinitely complex. Since there is as yet no way to study the complex interactions that occur between chemical constituents, they are studied in isolation.

Second, if one is not well versed in the language, it is difficult to understand the (albeit limited) conclusions drawn by this approach. Much confusion and misinformation has arisen as a result.

Still, the constituent-based understanding of aromatherapy has brought much to the field — certainly in terms of safety; namely, we now have specific dilutions that have been tested for efficacy and safety, and we have learned a great deal about contraindications for the oils. The main constituent of each oil is listed in the chart at the end of this chapter, and a more thorough exploration of this subject can be found in References (see page 264).

Measuring the Effects of Aromatherapy

Investigating one constituent taken from a plant that contains thousands, if not millions, of compounds is by definition reductionist and can never reveal the complete picture, nor can it describe all the medical possibilities of a particular essential oil.

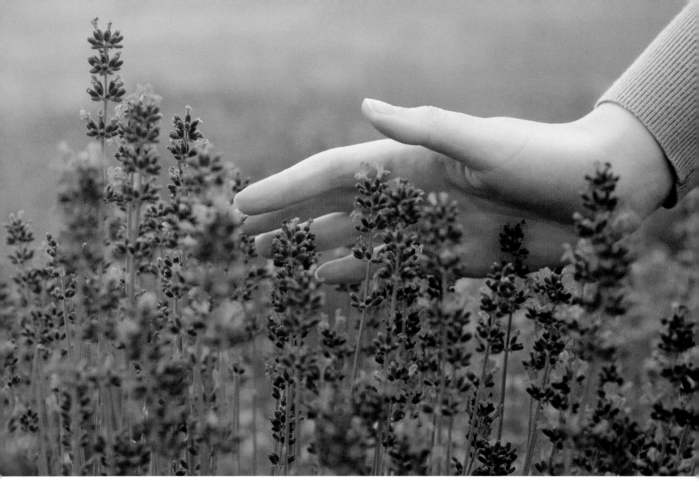

Essential Oils: Interacting with Human Physiology

Our bodies have been designed to keep the outside world out, but controlled pathways to the interior do exist (obviously, or we could not consume the food that we rely on to rebuild our bodies). If we want to bring an essential oil into the body, we can do so in several different ways.

Inhalation

Here, we focus on why inhalation might be the most appropriate method of application.

It is pretty clear that scent molecules are meant to be enjoyed or they wouldn't be capable of generating feel-good endorphins and dopamine, for example. The euphoric oils, such as jasmine and other florals, are called heady for a reason — one intoxicating whiff and we can feel transformed by their beauty. They paint their story on the emotional canvas of our interior life, enriching our appreciation of beauty through scent. Inhalation is a highly effective way of accessing and balancing many systems, including the respiratory, for example, and the oxygen it brings us, as well as the circulatory system as it moves our blood.

As we saw in Chapter 1, "Understanding Chinese Medicine and Its Therapies," the relationship between qi and the blood is described as interdependent. The metaphor heard most commonly is that of the bus and the driver. The blood carries the qi around the body, while the qi drives the blood around the body. It goes without saying that if there is a problem with either, both suffer. The relationship between the respiratory and circulatory systems is similarly interdependent. The two exist to serve each other: the blood carries the oxygen around and respiration drives the movement of blood. When an essential oil molecule is inhaled, first it affects the respiratory, but it is soon found in the bloodstream.

Caution When Inhaling

Many people are extremely sensitive to inhaled scents, whether from natural or synthetic sources. When introducing essential oils for the first time to a person with known sensitivities or respiratory conditions, it is imperative that the process be closely monitored and to proceed with caution. In some cases, it may be necessary to quickly open and close the bottle some distance away — a few feet (meters) or so — and wait for a minute to see if the scent molecules cause any distress. Never apply an oil to a sensitive person without first testing for reactions, regardless of the application method (inhaled or topical, for example).

When to Use Inhalation

In general terms, when there is congestion in the upper part of the body, consider administering essential oils via inhalation. Congestion can be an indication of inflammation, phlegm stagnation (such as with chronic bronchitis) or blood stagnation, a term that describes conditions such as coronary artery disease. Simply put, when there is too little movement in the head or chest, inhalation is appropriate.

Keep in mind that even if the primary application is via a different delivery method — topical (on the skin), for example — a great deal of scent is still volatilizing into the air. In fact, an inhalation component accompanies many different types of application, just from opening the bottle! This is because essential oil molecules are very small. The numbers we use to assign molecular weight really only give us a frame of reference, because it is nearly impossible to imagine the weight, or mass, of a substance so light that its nature is to escape its source and drift through the air. The tiny size of the molecules also allows them to easily enter the blood through the skin.

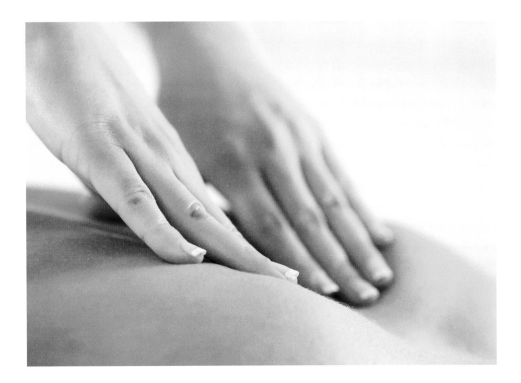

External

Skin

The process described in Chapter 4 of this book, "Acupressure and Aromatherapy for Conditions," focuses on applying the oils to the skin, over specific acupressure points. The main application technique is on the skin for several important reasons.

The skin is a deeply underappreciated organ. It is our biggest organ by far and performs the most important role of any organ — maintaining integrity. The skin keeps us whole, holding in our other organs and offering a contained environment designed to support the physiological functions that take place both within and throughout the skin. It also provides a barrier of immunity between us and the billions of substances we encounter every day.

In addition to providing a physical obstacle, the skin provides a perfect milieu for the surface bacteria we carry around. It is estimated that the average human carries nearly 5 pounds (2.2 kg) of bacteria on the skin, most of which are working to keep pathogenic bacteria — those known to cause disease — from entering our system via the skin. These beneficial microbial populations maintain a healthy environment through a complex set of checks and balances to ensure homeodynamics, the constantly changing interrelatedness of body components that works to maintain equilibrium overall. For thousands of years, this was a fairly routine process. With the advent of scientific advances, however, our native microbial populations have been changing and interacting differently.

Germm Theory

The concept of the germ was postulated several centuries ago. In 1675, Antonie van Leeuwenhoek, a Dutch tradesman and lens maker widely accepted as the man who invented the microscope, looked at a drop of rain and discovered it was teeming with tiny creatures he called "animalcules" (tiny animals). The realization that we are surrounded by microscopic life changed modern science. It is hard to believe from our modern vantage point that the concept of germ theory, for example, was still largely unknown until the mid-19th century.

The wholesale acceptance of the idea that germs cause illness has led to an overly hygienic world where our native flora are constantly being thrown out of balance. The use of antibacterial soaps, for example, further disrupt the homeodynamic bacterial layer. The rise in eczema, dermatitis and autoimmune diseases can be traced in part to extreme hygienic practices.

This is true of our inner "skin" as well. Mammals are basically shaped like a doughnut; that is, the outer skin is connected with our inner skin — the lining of our digestive system — to form a continuous barrier to the outside world. The bacterial load in our gut is perhaps even more important for protecting us from invading pathogens.

Touch

The skin has many physiological functions as well. The one we tend to think of first is touch, that most lovely sensation so necessary for human beings. Many studies have revealed the importance of touch for humans to function properly; "hug" studies, for example, show that rubbing or patting the back releases oxytocin, the same chemical that is triggered when babies cry and results in the letdown of mom's milk. In other words, rubbing stimulates our desire to nurture.

The skin is capable of responding to the lightest touches, so that the wind caressing our skin can evoke an emotional response, depending upon what we associate with the feeling. Consider this experience I had several years ago:

> *I remember it was quite windy while I was hiking up to a high alpine meadow in Switzerland. The constant buffeting was wearing me out, and despite the natural beauty surrounding me, my flagging energy was occupying my attention. As I hiked the last switchback on the trail, the wind suddenly died away completely just as the most incredible vista unfolded in front of me. As I sat there, catching my breath, the tiniest breeze played in my hair, tickled my face, bringing with it the scent of wildflowers and evergreens. My exhaustion fell away and happiness flooded me. To this day, when tiny zephyrs tease at my perception, I can instantly recall that sensation of awe and peace. On the other hand, a buffeting gale reminds me of the exhaustion of the trail that predominated just before I arrived at the meadow.*

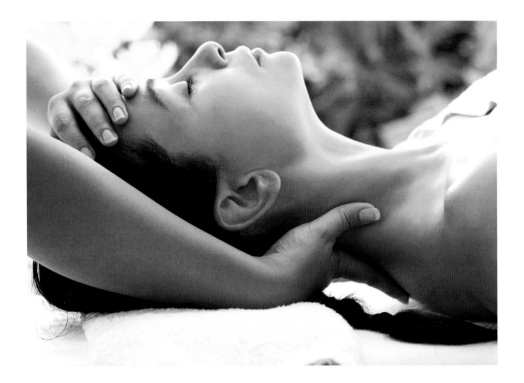

Acupressure is a type of touch. Both the act of palpating for the point and the act of applying pressure are stimulating physiological functions that contribute to health (see directions for acupressure, page 21). When combined with aromatherapy, the effects are dynamically enhanced through inhalation and transdermal absorption, described in this chapter.

Temperature Control

The skin also plays a large role in temperature regulation. Imagine ancient humans, back from a long day of hunting woolly mammoths, standing in the entrance to the communal cave, gazing out over the tundra. As their sweat cools, a frigid Arctic wind passes by, instantly chilling the drying sweat.

This kind of direct communication from the outside speaks to thermoreceptors in our skin, which signal the rate of discharge of warmth to slow dramatically. The cold receptors become less active, as the message has already been received, and the sudoriferous (sweat) glands dramatically slow their output in an effort to retain heat. Skeletal muscles start to make tiny movements — the shivers — generating warmth in an attempt to maintain a state of homeodynamis.

Hopefully, by this time, our Stone Age friend has moved deeper into the cave to stand by the fire that perpetually burns in the center. In modern times, all of this may occur without us even being aware of it, but in the Paleolithic world, it was imperative that these external messages be recognized or the consequences could be dire.

Both acupressure and essential oils can be very helpful for regulating temperature. Take the two examples here on how they work together to address a condition: Essential oils high in aldehydes, for example basil, are antipyretic (cooling), and several acupressure points are also classically used to reduce a fever; warming oils like ginger or black pepper can help poor circulation to the extremities, and adding very small amounts of these oils to a bath can increase core temperature fast.

Delivery through the Skin

The skin was once believed to be an extremely limited pathway because it was primarily understood to be a barrier. We now know that it makes an excellent delivery system, with some key limitations. This process, called transdermal absorption, allows us to draw nutrients and other substances into the bloodstream. To understand transdermal absorption, we need to take a brief look at skin physiology.

The skin is made up of several layers. The basic divisions are:

- the epidermis, or outermost layer
- the dermis, where most of the functional structures, such as nerves and blood vessels, are found
- the subcutaneous tissue

Semi-Waterproof Barrier

The outermost layer of the epidermis, called the stratum corneum, is made up of cells high in keratin, a substance that helps maintain skin hydration by reducing moisture loss — in effect, keratin contributes to the creation of a semi-waterproof barrier.

The outermost layer of the epidermis — the stratum corneum — is high in keratin. This hydrophobic ("water-fearing") layer sits on top of a hydrophilic ("water-loving") layer, which readily accepts water and water-based substances.

The more the cells of the stratum corneum are exposed to water, the looser the junctions between them become. The wrinkles we get on our fingers after a long soak in the tub result from water being absorbed into the skin, across the stratum corneum, to the water-loving layer beneath. Studies have shown that hydrated skin is up to three times more likely to absorb substances across its surface.

Of course, if there is a way to bring substances in through the skin, there must also be a way to get waste out. Our bodies are capable of clearing waste through the skin, and essential oils can play an effective role here. When the other primary organs of elimination (colon, liver and lungs, for example) become overloaded and less capable of removing toxins, the skin will pick up the extra work to relieve the burden.

Removing Toxins

The skin is an emmunctory organ; that is, an organ of elimination. It is both a primary emmunctory — clearing metabolic waste via sweating — and can act as a secondary emmunctory when other organs are overloaded and can no longer remove toxins on their own.

Oils such as peppermint (*Mentha piperita*) or rosemary (*Rosemarinus officinalis*) help the skin act as a secondary emmunctory by opening the pores, thus helping the body rid itself of metabolic wastes.

Clearly, topical applications of essential oils can be extremely effective. For more information on how to take advantage of the ways in which essential oils are known to help certain conditions when applied to specific sites, see Chapter 4, "Acupressure and Aromatherapy for Conditions."

Internal

Suppository, Pessary, Douche, Enema

While all skin surfaces provide a potential entry site for essential oils, certain tissues in the body, such as mucous membranes, are particularly receptive to transdermal absorption. The sinuses and throat are effectively treated with aromatherapy, and both the vagina and anus are rich in blood vessels that readily absorb scent molecules. Further, the urinary system is intricately linked to both the oxygen and the blood, so this is another system that benefits from transdermal absorption of the oils. These types of delivery methods are underutilized in North America, even though they were once a primary mode of home treatment. In many parts of the world, these methods are still widely used, however, as the tissues of the vagina and anus are perfectly designed to benefit from EOs. Mucous membranes easily absorb the benefits directly, and the concentrated blood vessels of the anus will quickly transfer molecules directly into the bloodstream. (See How to Use Essential Oils, page 103, for more on appropriate essential oils and dilutions.)

Adding tiny amounts of EOs to a highly mucilaginous decoction, like marshmallow, to use as an enema (applied into the rectum), will not only slow absorption of the EO, but also soothe and protect irritated mucous membranes. A pessary made from slippery elm inserted into the vagina will heal vaginal irritation quite nicely on its own, but adding a drop of rose geranium to address the fungal load is smart and effective — rose geranium, uniquely, is not as antibacterial as some essential oils but works beautifully against fungus infections. It is also less likely to wipe out the native bacterial populations of the vagina; that is, our allies working hard to return balance.

Oral Ingestion

This is an area of contention in the essential oil world. In some parts of the world, essential oils are regularly ingested, and in other countries it is strictly forbidden. Ironically, we ingest essential oils every time we eat — much of the flavor of food comes from the essential oils found in whole food impacting our sense of smell. What would an orange taste like if we couldn't smell it? Think of all the herbs we cook with daily, and how many of them play an important role in the aromatherapy kit.

Admittedly, essential oils are super-concentrated, and like any dense healing substance, following dosage directions is key. It might be helpful to consider the ideas behind homeopathy — minute amounts of substances can alter a person's state both subtly and in a grand manner. This is similar to synthetic pharmaceuticals — many work with the subtle shifting of tiny amounts of hormones or neurotransmitters, and large doses or overuse can lead to dire consequences, in particular sensitization.

What is Sensitization?

Sensitization may result from overexposure to essential oils (EOs), so that an oil that was once tolerated now causes reactions in the user. The good news is we know that tiny concentrations of EOs often result in the most effective health outcomes. For example, one drop of peppermint (*Mentha piperita*) essential oil is often enough to reduce digestive upset and is commonly prescribed for both IBD (inflammatory bowel disease, page 158) and some symptoms of GERD (page 192). It is important to note, however, that drinking a cup of peppermint (or ginger or fennel or orange peel) tea may be just as effective as using the oil.

From my perspective, ingesting essential oils internally can be an incredibly effective protocol, if used wisely. In most cases, it may be best reserved for serious diseases, both chronic and acute, or as a later intervention following more gentle treatments. However, a treatise on the internal use of essential oils is beyond the scope of this book.

Any substance that enters the body will eventually — usually sooner than later — enter the liver to be attached to a variety of different liver enzymes. Ingested essential oils are treated as potentially toxic, as are the foods we regularly eat since that is the default response of liver physiology. If the goal is to treat the gut or the liver, then ingestion might be the most appropriate delivery mechanism. If the target area is further down the system, then consider a different route, such as a topical application for athlete's foot or rectal treatments for the lower bowel.

Storage and Efficacy of Essential Oils

Many essential oils are extremely reactive; in particular, the oils categorized as high in aldehydes will readily oxidize and are easily destroyed by light. Because so many of the oils mentioned in this book are reactive, just to be safe, *store all of your EOs in a dark, cool place.* If you have room in the fridge, store your oils there. With some, you will need to think ahead and remove them from the fridge in advance of using them, since some oils — vetiver (*Vetiveria zizanoides*), for example — will thicken if they get cold.

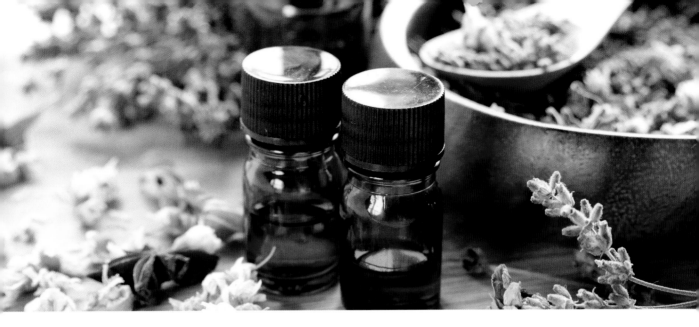

Another option is to be selective: research which oils most easily oxidize and ensure that they are always kept cool and out of the light. This is only necessary for the mother bottles; that is, the bottles of undiluted EOs. Any blends should be made in small amounts, with the intention of using them up in short order. Two-dram bottles are a good place to start, not only to avoid oxidation but to test out blends. It is a good idea to start with very small bottles for mixing. In a 2-dram bottle, which holds approximately 60 drops, at least 45 drops will be carrier oil, resulting in less waste of precious essential oils. If you decide to try a different combination, there is less waste.

How to Use Essential Oils

The chart starting on page 109 is a compilation of information I have gathered over the last 15 years of using essential oils, personally and later clinically. The information comes from a variety of sources, such as various books and colleagues that have contributed so much to my understanding. In fact, any body of knowledge is the accumulation of thousands of years of recorded history.

In the spirit of encouraging further studies, I assign credit to the following scholars as starting points for most of the information in the following pages.

Safety info: *Essential Oil Safety*, by Robert Tisserand and Rodney Young, is required reading when working with oils. Tisserand's knowledge of aromatherapy is widely respected and matched by his proficiency as a scientist. The book is the definitive collection of studies the authors used in determining safety levels and presents an in-depth chemical analysis of each oil. When the authors do not agree with the safety levels established by these studies, they offer a clear explanation. The section detailing the constituents is unparalleled. Many of my dilution suggestions come from early editions of this book.

Western medical aromatherapy indications and actions:

In *L'Aromathérapie Exactemente* by Pierre Franchomme and Daniel Pénoël, the authors present the medical science of essential oils and aromatherapy. This book introduced many aromatherapists to the concept of categorizing the oils by the actions ascribed to the primary chemical constituents.

Chemistry: Kurt Schnaubelt's *Advanced Aromatherapy* is an excellent introduction to the broader constituent-based categorization set forth by Franchomme and Pénoël. In addition, Sue Clarke's excellent *Essential Chemistry for Aromatherapy* is a first-rate primer on the basic chemistry concepts of essential oils — clear, concise and accessible. And, of course, *Essential Oil Safety* by Tisserand and Young also helps here.

Nature: This category we explore later refers to the temperature, direction and qualities of the oils from a Chinese Medicine perspective. Most of this information comes from testing involving the use of sense organs, also known as organoleptic testing, done by me and my students. I also consulted Dr. Heiner Fruehauf, my mentor and the founder of the Classical Chinese Medicine department at the National University of Natural Medicine in Portland.

Properties of Essential Oils: Chart Categories Explained

The chart of essential oils (pages 109 to 127) has the following information listed for each entry:

Plant Name *(Latin binomial):* plant part used

Dilution: Maximum dilution for safe use

Warning: Any warning or caution pertaining to use of the oil

Actions: The physiologic actions of the essential oil

Primary Compounds: A listing of the primary chemical compounds found in the essential oil

CM Nature: The essential oil's nature according to Chinese Medicine categories

Conditions: Conditions for which the oil is suggested in this book

Glossary: For more information for terms that are unfamiliar or specialized in the chart, refer to the Glossary on page 262.

Maximum Dilution for Use

To achieve the proper dilution, use these proportions:

0.5% dilution = 2–3 drops of essential oil per ounce (28 g) of base oil or other carrier

1% dilution = 5 drops of essential oil per ounce (28 g) of base oil or other carrier

2% dilution = 10 drops of essential oil per ounce (28 g) of base oil or other carrier

2.5% dilution = 15 drops of essential oil per ounce (28 g) of base oil or other carrier

3% dilution = 20 drops of essential oil per ounce (28 g) of base oil or other carrier

4% dilution = 25 drops of essential oil per ounce (28 g) of base oil or other carrier

5% dilution = 30 drops of essential oil per ounce (28 g) of base oil or other carrier

10% dilution = 60 drops of essential oil per ounce (28 g) of base oil or other carrier

Warning/Caution

Note specific warnings listed. Some oils are **photosensitizing**, for example, meaning they may increase the damage to the skin caused by sunlight. Phototoxic oils are noted in the chart.

Many people are extremely **sensitive to inhaled scents**, whether from natural or synthetic sources. When introducing essential oils for the first time to a person with known sensitivities or respiratory conditions, it is imperative that the process be closely monitored and to proceed with caution. In some cases, it may be necessary to quickly open and close the bottle some distance away — a few feet (meters) or so — and wait for a minute to see if the scent molecules cause any distress. Never apply an oil to a sensitive person without first testing for reactions, regardless of the application method (inhaled or topical, for example).

When working with **children or pregnant women**, be extra cautious, especially about dilutions. The correct dilution for children 5 to 10 years of age is 0.5% to 1%. For children under 10, it is recommended to purchase a specialized book on aromatherapy for children. This holds true for pregnant women as well — purchase a book on pregnancy and aromatherapy. According to Tisserand, the following oils should never be used in pregnancy: wormwood, rue, oak moss, French lavender (*Lavandula stoechas*), camphor, parsley seed, sage and hyssop (*Hyssopus officinalis*).

Finally, if there is a history of a **seizure disorder**, be extremely cautious when using essential oils, as they may trigger seizures — as described above, essential oils act primarily in the nervous and endocrine systems. There is no definitive list of oils that are likely to cause seizures, so always assume that any oil may be a seizure trigger.

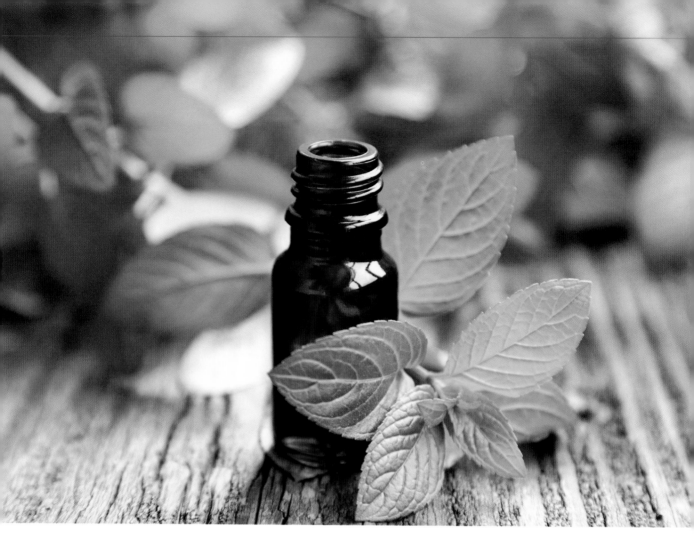

Primary Chemical Compounds

The two main classes that make up the aromatic compounds of plants are *hydrocarbons* and *oxygenated hydrocarbons*. Hydrocarbons are hard to group, as most have unique characteristics. The hydrocarbon groups found in essential oils are terpenes (monoterpenes, sesquiterpenes).

Oxygenated hydrocarbons make a compound less active, that is, less irritating. For example, monoterpene alcohols (monoterpenols), in general, have a reputation for being gentler. Other oxygenated compounds include: phenols, esters, lactones, aldehydes and ketones.

Monoterpenols:

Aromatherapists rely on the monoterpenols for being less irritating and broadly healing. Nearly all are antimicrobial, effective against bacteria, viruses and fungus. They offer immune support, and tend to relax the pulmonocirculatory system. Examples of monoterpenols include:

Linalool, found in thyme linalool
Citronellol, found in geranium
Menthol, found in peppermint

Sesquiterpenols:

Sesquiterpene alcohols (sesquiterpenols) have a reputation for helping with nerve and muscle dystonia (lack of tone), and are used to tonify circulation especially of the venous system. Some sesquiterpenols have more specific functions, like carotol, which is known to help regenerate liver tissue. Examples of sesquiterpenols include:

α-Bisabolol, found in German chamomile

α-Santalol, found in sandalwood

Carotol, found in carrot seed

Phenols:

Phenols are generally more stimulating. They are also known for their antimicrobial effects. Examples of phenols include:

Carvacrol, found in oregano

Eugenol, found in clove

Thymol, found in thyme thymol

Esters:

Esters are distinguished by their sweet, fruity scent and are generally very mild (non-reactive). They are also known for their antispasmodic effect. Examples of esters include:

Linalyl acetate, found in clary sage

Geranyl acetate, found in geranium

Ethers:

The majority of ethers from essential oils that we are interested in are phenylpropanoid ethers. They share many characteristics with the esters, despite being formed from phenols. Examples of phenylpropanoid ethers include:

(E)-Anethole, found in aniseed

Apiole, from parsley

Lactones:

Lactones form from esters; they are cooling and many are mucolytic and expectorant. A special class of lactones, coumarins, have anticoagulant properties and should be used with caution in individuals suffering from clotting disorders. Examples of lactones include:

Nepetalactone, found in catnip

Coumarin, found in the odor of new-mown hay

Bergapten, found in bergamot

Aldehydes:

Aldehydes are very reactive, and are known for being sedative and anti-inflammatory, antispasmodic and antiviral. Examples of aldeydes include:

Citral, found in melissa

Geranial, found in lemongrass

Ketones:

Ketones are generally cicatrisants and many are mucolytic. Examples of ketones include:

Pinocamphone, found in hyssop

Menthone, found in peppermint

Nature According to Chinese Categories

Some oils are astringent and tend to dry out a damp condition, while others draw moisture to a site to help lubricate and moisturize it, so the Nature category helps us understand whether the oil is encouraging moistening or drying. Another way to understand this is whether it is tonifying or relaxing to the tissue. Within the Nature category, the temperature and direction of the oil are also considered.

- **Temperature:** indicates the influence of the oil on the body. For warm conditions, it may be appropriate to use neutral to cooling oils, or it might be more effective to use warming oils to encourage the action the body is attempting to effect, like in a fever, for example.

- **Direction:** Does the oil move qi down or up? Or does it do both (circulating)? Does it encourage qi to move in (tonify) or out (protect)? For conditions where there is excess upward movement, such as vomiting or headache, will the oil help descend the excess upward movement? Most oils move in more than one way, however, so the primary direction is given.

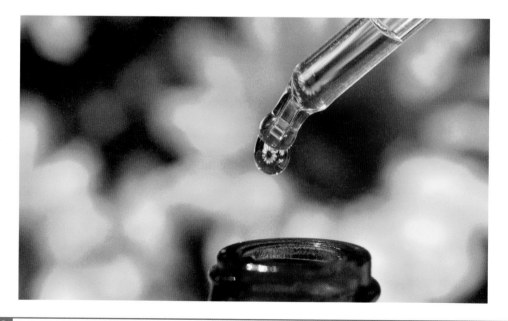

Properties of Essential Oils

Angelica *(Angelica archangelica):* root

Dilution: 0.5% dilution

Warning: The oil is phototoxic at higher concentrations. Even at the recommended dilution, do not expose the skin to direct sunlight for at least 12 hours. May be sensitizing.

Actions: The plant has a long history of use as a digestive aid. Carminative, sedative

Primary Compounds: Phellandrene; monoterpene

CM Nature: Warm, dry, circulating

Conditions: Addiction

Aniseed *(Pimpinella anisum):* seed

Dilution: 2% dilution

Warning: Safety studies suggest that this oil is contraindicated in pregnancy, breastfeeding, endometriosis, estrogen-dependent cancers or for use on children under 5. It is not available over the counter in France because of certain constituents that may be problematic.

Actions: Antiseptic, antispasmodic, carminative, cardiac tonic, cholagogue, estrogen-like, respiratory tonic, vermifuge

Primary Compounds: (E)-anethole; phenylpropanoid ether

CM Nature: Neutral, dry, descending

Conditions: Bloating

Basil *(Ocimum basilicum):* leaves

Dilution: 1% dilution

Warning: Avoid in pregnancy. May be mildly sensitizing to the skin (animal studies). For sensitive individuals, it is best to start with *Ocimum basilicum* L., as this is the mildest form and least irritating to the skin. The L stands for linalool.

Actions: Neuroregulatory effects; antispasmodic; anti-inflammatory, especially resulting from infection; venous decongestant, especially of the vena cava; respiratory; prostate; veins, antiviral; antibacterial

Primary Compounds: In basil linalool, linalool; monoterpenol

CM Nature: Warm, dry, descending, inward (tonifying)

Conditions: Aphthous ulcers (mouth sores), bowel incontinence, adhesive capsulitis (frozen shoulder), common cold, constipation, diarrhea, indigestion, insufficient lactation, sciatica, tinnitus (ringing in the ears)

Birch *(Betula lenta):* bark

Dilution: 2% dilution

Warning: Possible drug interactions (check prescriptions). Contraindicated for those with salicylate allergies. Avoid in GERD. Avoid in pregnancy and breastfeeding.

Actions: Antispasmodic, anti-inflammatory, hepatostimulant

Primary Compounds: Methyl salicylate; esters

CM Nature: Cool, dry, descending

Conditions: Headache, torticollis (neck spasm, stiff neck)

Black pepper *(Piper nigrum):* fruit

Dilution: 2%–4% dilution

Warning: Oxidation — needs to be refrigerated

Actions: Anticatarrhal; expectorant; mucolytic; stimulates digestive enzymes; analgesic, especially toothache; febrifuge

Primary Compounds: β-caryophyllene; sesquiterpene

CM Nature: Hot, dry, out

Conditions: Adhesive capsulitis (frozen shoulder), circulation, halitosis (bad breath) due to tooth decay, pain of all kinds, phlegm, rhinitis (runny or stuffy nose), thyroid imbalance, subacute trigeminal neuralgia (facial nerve pain)

Carrot seed *(Daucus carota):* seed

Dilution: 2%–4% dilution

Warning: Contraindicated in pregnancy and lactation

Actions: Hypertensive; detoxifying, especially to the liver; hepatoregenerative; somewhat anticoagulant

Primary Compounds: Carotol; sesquiterpene

CM Nature: Neutral, moistening, ascending

Conditions: Hepatitis and other viral infections of the liver, hiccup, menopausal symptoms, urinary incontinence, varicosities

Chamomile species

German chamomile *(Matricaria recutita):* aerial parts

Dilution: 4% dilution

Warning: Possible drug interactions (check prescriptions). May be allergenic.

Actions: Digestive tonic, anti-inflammatory, cicatrisant, antiallergenic, decongestant, hormone-like, antispasmodic

Primary Compounds: α-bisabolol oxide A; sesquiterpene

CM Nature: Neutral to cooling, moistening, circulating (tonifying)

Conditions: Eczema, conjunctivitis (pinkeye)

Blue chamomile *(Tanacetum annuum):* aerial parts

Dilution: 4% dilution

Warning: May be allergenic

Actions: Anti-inflammatory; antihistamine; antipruritic; antalgic, for back pain; sedative; hypotensive

Primary Compounds: α-bisabolol oxide A; sesquiterpene

CM Nature: Neutral to cooling, moistening, circulating (tonifying)

Conditions: Cough, nausea and vomiting, rhinitis (runny or stuffy nose), skin blemishes, bleeding gums, eczema

Roman chamomile *(Anthemis nobilis):* aerial parts

Dilution: 4% dilution

Warning: None known. May be allergenic

Actions: Antispasmodic, anti-inflammatory, CNS depressant, antiparasitic

Primary Compounds: Esters

CM Nature: Neutral to warming, moistening, ascending (moving)

Conditions: Hiccup, insufficient lactation, Raynaud syndrome, osteoarthritis

Cinnamon *(Cinnamomum verum):* bark

Dilution: 0.5% dilution

Warning: Possible drug interactions, especially anticoagulants (check prescriptions). Contraindicated in pregnancy and breastfeeding, but excellent for postpartum moms; irritating to mucus membranes; avoid with bleeding disorders.

Actions: Anti-infection agent, antibacterial, antiparasitic, antiseptic, preservative, anesthetizing, aphrodisiac, anticoagulant, regulates blood sugar, stimulates menstruation by increasing uterine contractions, respiratory tonic, tonic to sympathetic nervous system

Primary Compounds: E-cinnamaldehyde; aldehyde

CM Nature: Hot, dry, descending/circulating, inward (tonifying)

Conditions: Irregular menstruation (excessive bleeding), menopausal symptoms, nocturnal enuresis (bedwetting), hypothyroidism, vertigo, common cold, diarrhea, fungal infections of the nails

Clary sage *(Salvia sclarea):* aerial parts

Dilution: 2% dilution

Warning: Sensitivity warning: 0.25% max for sensitive individuals. Avoid in estrogen-dominant imbalances. According to leading practitioner Jeffrey Yuen, alcohol use is a contraindication.

Actions: Estrogen-like, aphrodisiac, regulates blood sugar, antihypercholesterolemia, anti-infection agent, antibacterial, antifungal, antispasmodic, may reduce likelihood of seizures, nervous system tonic

Primary Compounds: Linalyl acetate; ester

CM Nature: Cooling, moistening, ascending/circulating

Conditions: Menopausal symptoms, leukorrhea (vaginal discharge) due to yeast infection, irregular menstruation

Clove *(Syzygium aromaticum,* aka *Eugenia caryophyllata):* buds

Dilution: 0.5% dilution

Warning: Possible drug interactions, especially anticoagulants — avoid with bleeding disorders (check prescriptions). Irritating to mucous membranes, including gums. If using for gum pain, limit use to a day or two. Avoid in pregnancy and breastfeeding and for children.

Actions: Wide-spectrum antibiotic, antiviral, antifungal, antiparasitic, antiseptic, styptic

Primary Compounds: Eugenol; phenylpropane

CM Nature: Hot, drying, inward

Conditions: Aphthous ulcers (mouth sores), diarrhea, fungal infections (thrush), toothache

Cypress *(Cupressus sempervirens):* leaves and branches

Dilution: 2%–4% dilution

Warning: Oxidation — needs to be refrigerated

Actions: Venous decongestant, lymphatic decongestant, reduces prostatic inflammation, antibacterial, effective against mycobacterium; tonic, especially to the nervous system

Primary Compounds: Monoterpenes, especially α-pinene

CM Nature: Cooling, moistening (by redistributing fluids), circulating (in)

Conditions: Angina; asthma due to upper respiratory infection; respiratory bacterial infections; edema, especially of the upper body; nocturnal enuresis (bedwetting); prostatitis; skin blemishes with excess oil production; varicosities; vertigo

Eucalyptus species

Eucalyptus citriodora: leaves

Dilution: 10% (up to 20%) dilution

Warning: Caution with children under 10. May lead to skin sensitization.

Actions: Anti-inflammatory, antirheumatic, sedative, antihypertensive, pain reducer, anti-infection agent, somewhat antispasmodic

Primary Compounds: 1,8-cineole; monoterpene

CM Nature: Warming, drying, up and out

Conditions: Eczema, viral infections of the liver, rheumatoid arthritis

Eucalyptus globulus: leaves

Dilution: 10% (up to 20%) dilution

Warning: Caution with children under 10. May lead to skin sensitization.

Actions: Expectorant, mucolytic, antimicrobial, antifungal, antiviral, antiseptic

Primary Compounds: 1,8-cineole; monoterpene

CM Nature: Warming, drying, up and out

Conditions: Acute bronchitis, common cold in adults, cough, halitosis (bad breath) due to sinus infection, phlegm, viral infections

Eucalyptus radiata: leaves

Dilution: 10% (up to 20%) dilution

Warning: Caution with children under 10; Despite being an appropriate EO to use with children, use caution with children under 10 — use a lower (2%) dilution. May lead to skin sensitization.

Actions: Antimicrobial, antifungal, antiviral, antiseptic, expectorant, mucolytic, anti-inflammatory

Primary Compounds: 1,8-cineole; monoterpene

CM Nature: Warming, drying, up and out

Conditions: Common cold in children, viral infections in children

---

Fennel *(Foeniculum vulgare):* seed

Dilution: 2% dilution

Warning: Possible drug interactions, especially hormone therapies. Avoid with bleeding disorders. Contraindicated during pregnancy and breastfeeding, although fennel tea is excellent for helping with milk production.

Actions: Estrogen-like, emmenagogue, galactogogue, cholagogue, antispasmodic, carminative, appetite stimulant; tonic, especially respiratory and cardiac

Primary Compounds: (E)-anethole; phenylpropanoid ether

CM Nature: Warming, drying, in and down

Conditions: GERD (acid reflux), bloating, constipation, diarrhea, edema, halitosis (bad breath) due to gastrointestinal disturbance, acute hepatitis A, indigestion, insufficient lactation, nausea and vomiting

---

Fir *(Abies alba):* needles

Dilution: 2% dilution

Warning: Oxidation — needs to be refrigerated

Actions: Antiseptic, mucolytic

Primary Compounds: Camphene; monoterpene

CM Nature: Cooling, moistening (redistributes fluids), up

Conditions: Chronic bronchitis, phlegm

Frankincense *(Boswellia carteri):* resin tears (solidified resin)

Dilution: 2% dilution

Warning: Oxidation — needs to be refrigerated

Actions: Mucolytic, expectorant, cicatrisant (generates new skin)

Primary Compounds: α-pinene; monoterpene

CM Nature: Neutral to warming, neutral to drying, up and out (for example, if there is damp in the lungs, it will help move that moisture up and out through the mucolytic, expectorant properties, but it will also moisten the skin when applied topically, and the movement is up and out as it is calling moisture to the surface)

Conditions: Anxiety disorder, asthma, bipolar disorder, bowel incontinence, depression, eczema, menopausal symptoms (vaginal dryness, decreased libido), toothache, varicosities

....

Geranium, rose *(Pelargonium graveolens):* leaves

Dilution: 5% dilution

Warning: Possible drug interactions (check prescriptions)

Actions: Antispasmodic, anti-inflammatory, pain reducer, hemostatic, lymph and venous tonic, stimulates hepatic activity, antifungal, stimulates nervous activity in peripheral neuropathies

Primary Compounds: Citronellol; monoterpene alcohol

CM Nature: Neutral, down and inward (tonifying)

Conditions: Fungal infections of all kinds (vaginal, thrush, skin), menopausal symptoms

....

Ginger *(Zingiber officinale):* root

Dilution: 2%–4% dilution

Warning: None known

Actions: Digestive tonic, carminative, pain reliever, expectorant and mucolytic

Primary Compounds: Zingiberene; sesquiterpene

CM Nature: Hot, dry, circulating

Conditions: Nausea of all kinds, pain of all kinds, phlegm, prostatitis, rhinitis (runny or stuffy nose), trigeminal neuralgia (facial nerve pain), ulcers

Grapefruit *(Citrus paradisi):* peel

Dilution: 2% dilution

Warning: Oxidation — needs to be refrigerated. Phototoxicity — avoid direct sun for at least 8 hours after using.

Actions: Antiseptic, especially for airborne microbes

Primary Compounds: (+)-limonene; monoterpene

CM Nature: Neutral to cooling, drying, down

Conditions: GERD (acid reflux), addiction (nervous eating), edema, toothache

----

Helichrysum *(Helichrysum italicum):* aerial parts

Dilution: 2%–4% dilution

Warning: None known

Actions: Anticoagulant, venous decongestant, reduces bruising, stimulates hepatic regeneration, mucolytic, expectorant, antispasmodic, cicatrisant

Primary Compounds: α-pinene; monoterpene

CM Nature: Neutral temperature, neutral nature, circulating direction. This oil moves in and out, up and down and is excellent for moving stagnation.

Conditions: Addiction (nicotine), adhesive capsulitis (frozen shoulder), angina, eczema, bipolar disorder, bruising, carpal tunnel syndrome, cystitis (urinary tract infection), depression, epicondylitis (tennis/golfer's elbow), hepatitis, irregular menstruation, mastitis, plantar fasciitis, pain of all kinds, Raynaud syndrome, sciatica, trigeminal neuralgia (facial nerve pain), urinary incontinence, varicosities

----

Holy basil *(Ocimum tenuiflorum,* aka *Ocimum sanctum L.):* leaves

Dilution: 0.5% dilution

Warning: Possible drug interactions (check prescriptions)

Actions: Antispasmodic; nervous system tonic; anti-inflammatory; pain reducer; venous decongestant; reduces prostatic congestion; antibacterial, especially against staph species

Primary Compounds: Estragole; phenylpropanoid ether

CM Nature: Warming, drying, up

Conditions: Mental addictions, depression, rhinitis (runny or stuffy nose)

Hyssop *(Hyssopus officinalis* var. *decumbens,* note variety): aerial parts

Dilution: 2%–4% dilution

Warning: Oxidation — needs to be refrigerated

Actions: Mucolytic; expectorant; reduces frequency and severity of asthma symptoms (see Warning/Caution box); anti-inflammatory; bacteriocidal, especially against strep species; effective against *Candida albicans*; viricidal; tonic for central nervous system

Primary Compounds: Eugenol; phenylpropane; pinocamphone

CM Nature: Neutral to cooling, drying, down, out

Conditions: Allergies, asthma, phlegm, rhinitis (runny or stuffy nose)

....

Inula *(Inula graveolens):* flowers

Dilution: 2% dilution

Warning: None known

Actions: Antiseptic, anti-inflammatory, antispasmodic, cough suppressant, strongly mucolytic, may help regulate cardiac rhythm

Primary Compounds: Bornyl acetate; ester

CM Nature: Neutral to warm, up

Conditions: Allergies, bronchitis, rhinitis (runny or stuffy nose)

....

Juniper berry *(Juniperus communis):* berry

Dilution: 2%%–4% dilution

Warning: Oxidation — needs to be refrigerated

Actions: Expectorant, mucolytic, diuretic, antiseptic, effective for reducing rheumatic pain

Primary Compounds: α-pinene; monoterpene

CM Nature: Warming, moistening (redistributes fluids), down/circulating

Conditions: Arthritis, specifically osteoarthritis of the lower body, especially knees; cystitis (urinary tract infection), especially with a history of kidney infection; edema, especially due to diabetes

Laurel *(Laurus nobilis):* leaves

Dilution: 0.5% dilution

Warning: Caution with children under 10. May lead to skin sensitization.

Actions: Expectorant, mucolytic, antibacterial, antispasmodic, lymphatic decongestant, pain reducer

Primary Compounds: 1,8-cineole; monoterpene

CM Nature: Neutral to cooling, moistening (redistributes fluids), in/out circulation (tonifying/clearing)

Conditions: Aphthous ulcers (mouth sores), plantar fasciitis

Lavender *(Lavandula angustifolia):* aerial parts

Dilution: 2%–10%

Warning: None known

Actions: Antispasmodic; nervous system equilibrator; reduces muscular contracture; anti-inflammatory; antibacterial, especially against staph species; cicatrisant

Primary Compounds: Linalool; monoterpene

CM Nature: Neutral to cooling, moisturizing, up/systemic circulation

Conditions: Alopecia (hair loss), anxiety disorder, bacterial infection, conjunctivitis (pinkeye), constipation, diarrhea, headache, mastitis

---

Lemon *(Citrus limon):* peel

Dilution: 1% dilution

Warning: Oxidation — needs to be refrigerated. The oil is phototoxic at higher concentrations. Even at the recommended dilution, do not expose the skin to direct sunlight for at least 12 hours.

Actions: Antibacterial, antiviral, antiseptic, may help regulate hyperactive pain response, increases microcirculation, litholitic (helps break up stones such as gallstones or kidney stones), carminative

Primary Compounds: (+)-limonene; monoterpene

CM Nature: Cooling, drying, in

Conditions: Diffuse into sick rooms to reduce airborne bacteria; varicosities

Lemongrass *(Cymbopogon flexuosus):* aerial parts

Dilution: 0.5% dilution

Warning: Oxidation — needs to be refrigerated. Possible drug interactions (check prescriptions)

Actions: Digestive tonic, vasodilatory, anti-inflammatory, sedative

Primary Compounds: Geranial; aldehyde

CM Nature: Cooling, drying (disperses fluids), in

Conditions: Eczema, fungal infections (tinea), plantar fasciitis

Marjoram *(Origanum majorana):* leaves

Dilution: 2%–4% dilution

Warning: None known

Actions: Antibacterial, especially gram-positive bacteria; antiseptic; nervous system regulator, encouraging parasympathetic system, pain reducer; digestive system stimulant

Primary Compounds: Terpinen-4-ol; monoterpene

CM Nature: Neutral to cooling, drying, descending

Conditions: Spasmodic cough

Mastic *(Pistacia lentiscus):* gum

Dilution: 5%–10% dilution

Warning: None known

Actions: Vein and lymphatic decongestant, reduces prostatic congestion

Primary Compounds: α-pinene; monoterpene

CM Nature: Warm, drying, up

Conditions: Stomach ulcer

Melissa *(Melissa officinalis):* aerial parts

Dilution: 0.5% dilution

Warning: Oxidation — needs to be refrigerated. Possible drug interactions (check prescriptions). Caution in sensitive individuals and children under 2

Actions: Sedative, nervous system equilibrator, litholitic, anti-inflammatory, strongly antiviral

Primary Compounds: Geranial; aldehyde; citral

CM Nature: Cooling, drying, circulating

Conditions: Bipolar disorder; viral infections, especially herpes (cold sores)

Myrrh *(Commiphora molmol):* resin tears

Dilution: 2%–4% dilution

Warning: Avoid in pregnancy and breastfeeding

Actions: Antiviral; antiparasitic; parasiticidal, especially ascaris species; vulnerary; helps moderate thyroid function

Primary Compounds: Monoterpenes

CM Nature: Neutral, moistening, up/down communication

Conditions: Aphthous ulcer (mouth sores), eczema, toothache, viral infections of the gastrointestinal tract

---

Niaouli *(Melaleuca quinquenervia):* leaves

Dilution: 2%–4% dilution

Warning: None known

Actions: Antibacterial, antiparasitic, strongly antifungal, anti-inflammatory, mucolytic, expectorant, venous decongestant, litholitic, hormone-like

Primary Compounds: (E)-nerolidol; sesquiterpene

CM Nature: Neutral, drying (disperses fluids), down

Conditions: Nail fungus

Orange *(Citrus aurantium):* peel

Dilution: 5% dilution

Warning: Oxidation — needs to be refrigerated

Actions: Sedative, anti-inflammatory, circulatory stimulant

Primary Compounds: (+)-limonene; monoterpene

CM Nature: Cooling, drying, up to encourage down

Conditions: Common cold, cystitis (urinary tract infection), diarrhea, indigestion, insomnia, thyroid imbalance, ulcer, sleeplessness due to chronic disease

Oregano *(Origanum vulgare):* leaves

Dilution: 0.5%–1% dilution

Warning: Possible drug interactions (check prescriptions). Avoid in bleeding disorders. Avoid in pregnancy and breastfeeding

Actions: Antimicrobial, across the spectrum; analgesic

Primary Compounds: Carvacrol; monoterpene phenol

CM Nature: Neutral to cooling, drying, descending

Conditions: Bacterial infections, diarrhea due to infection, nocturnal enuresis (bedwetting) due to infection, prostatitis

Patchouli *(Pogostemon cablin):* leaves

Dilution: 5%–10% dilution

Warning: Possible drug interactions (check prescriptions). Avoid in bleeding disorders

Actions: Decongestant, especially veins; anti-inflammatory; cell regenerating, especially skin; antiseptic; febrifuge; insectifuge

Primary Compounds: Patchouli alcohol; sesquiterpene

CM Nature: Warm, moisturizing, in

Conditions: Fungal infections of the skin (tinea)

Peppermint *(Mentha piperita):* leaves

Dilution: 2%–4% dilution

Warning: Avoid in severe liver or gallbladder disease. Mucous membrane irritant

Actions: Bactericidal; viricidal; fungicidal; vermicidal; tonic to many systems, including circulatory and digestive; carminative, mucolytic and expectorant; pain reducer; anti-inflammatory; hormone-like

Primary Compounds: (-)-menthol; monoterpenol; menthone

CM Nature: Cold/hot, drying, out (surface circulation)

Conditions: GERD (acid reflux), bloating, bowel incontinence, bronchitis, common cold, fungal infection, headache, hiccup, nausea and vomiting, phlegm, prostatitis, rhinitis (runny or stuffy nose), toothache, varicosities

Pine *(Pinus sylvestris):* needles

Dilution: 5% dilution

Warning: Oxidation — needs to be refrigerated

Actions: Hormone-like; endocrine tonic; nervous system tonic; antifungal; antiseptic; especially helpful with respiratory inflammatory conditions (bronchitis, asthma, sinusitis); may help with atherosclerotic plaques

Primary Compounds: α-pinene; monoterpene

CM Nature: Neutral, neutral, circulating (body-directed)

Conditions: Anxiety disorder, acute bronchitis, cough, phlegm, sore throat, thyroid imbalance

---

Ravintsara *(Cinnamomum camphora):* leaves

Dilution: 1% dilution

Warning: Oxidation — needs to be refrigerated. Estragole content may be carcinogenic.

Actions: Strongly antiviral, antibacterial, expectorant

Primary Compounds: Estragole; phenylpropanoid ether

CM Nature: Neutral, neutral, up/down circulation

Conditions: Bronchitis, common cold, cough, sore throat, laryngitis, respiratory viral infections

---

Rose otto *(Rosa damascena):* flowers

Dilution: 0.5% dilution

Warning: None known

Actions: Nervous system tonic, cicatrisant, aphrodisiac

Primary Compounds: (-)-citronellol; monoterpene

CM Nature: Warming, moisturizing, up

Conditions: Angina, anxiety disorder, bipolar disorder, bronchitis, bruising, depression, diarrhea, mental restlessness, mastitis, menopausal symptoms (vaginal dryness, decreased libido), Raynaud syndrome, toothache due to infection

Rosemary (*Rosmarinus officinalis):* leaves

Dilution: 2%–4% dilution

Warning: Caution with children under 10. May lead to skin sensitization

Actions: Mucolytic, expectorant, bacteriocidal, viricidal, antispasmodic, circulatory tonic, endocrine tonic, cicatrisant

Primary Compounds: 1,8-cineole; monoterpene

CM Nature: Warming, drying, up

Conditions: Adhesive capsulitis (frozen shoulder), alopecia (hair loss), angina, asthma, cough, diabetes, diarrhea, irregular menstruation, nocturnal enuresis (bedwetting), plantar fasciitis, Raynaud syndrome, rhinitis (runny or stuffy nose), sciatica, skin blemishes, subacute trigeminal neuralgia (facial nerve pain), varicosities, vertigo

---

Sage (*Salvia officinalis):* leaves

Dilution: 0.5% dilution

Warning: Ketones readily cross the blood–brain barrier and possibly lead to neurotoxicity. Avoid in pregnancy and breastfeeding

Actions: Mucolytic, expectorant, lipolytic, antibacterial, cicatrisant, reduces scar tissue

Primary Compounds: Camphor, α-thujone; monoterpene ketones

CM Nature: Neutral to warm, drying, in

Conditions: Rhinitis (runny or stuffy nose)

Spikenard (*Nardostachys jatamansi):* root

Dilution: 2%–4% dilution

Warning: None known

Actions: Sedative, venous tonic

Primary Compounds: Nardol; sesquiterpene

CM Nature: Warming, moisturizing, down

Conditions: Addiction, anxiety disorder, insomnia, tinnitus (ringing in the ears)

Spruce, black *(Picea mariana):* needles

Dilution: 1% dilution

Warning: Oxidation — needs to be refrigerated

Actions: Antispasmodic, anti-infection agent, antifungal, antiparasitic, anti-inflammatory, hormone-like, cortisone-like, neurotonic, antiseptic to airborne microbial agents

Primary Compounds: Bornyl acetate; ester

CM Nature: Warming, moisturizing, down to encourage up

Conditions: Bacterial infection, chronic fatigue, depression, exhaustion, nausea with exhaustion, phlegm, sore throat due to overuse, thyroid imbalance (hypothyroidism)

Tarragon *(Artemisia dracunculus):* leaves

Dilution: 0.5% dilution

Warning: Oxidation — needs to be refrigerated. Possible drug interactions (check prescriptions). Estragole content may be carcinogenic

Actions: Antispasmodic, especially esophageal spasm; anti-inflammatory; antibacterial; antiviral; may help with allergy symptoms

Primary Compounds: Estragole; phenylpropanoid ether

CM Nature: Warming, neutral, in

Conditions: GERD (acid reflux), hiccup, irregular menstruation

---

Tea tree *(Melaleuca alternifolia):* leaves

Dilution: 5%–15% dilution

Warning: Oxidation — needs to be refrigerated

Actions: Full-spectrum antimicrobial, anti-inflammatory, tonic to many systems, venous decongestant, cooling

Primary Compounds: Terpinen-4-ol; monoterpene

CM Nature: Neutral, drying (disperses fluids), down

Conditions: Fungal infection (tinea), leukorrhea (vaginal discharge), mastitis

Thyme species

Thymus vulgaris var. *linalool:* leaves

(milder version than thyme thymol)

Dilution: 2%–4% dilution

Warning: None known

Actions: Full-spectrum antimicrobial, cicatrisant

Primary Compounds: Linalool; monoterpene

CM Nature: Neutral, moisturizing, down

Conditions: Effective against the same conditions as thymol in early stages, in the elderly, or in children

Thymus vulgaris var. *thymol:* leaves

Dilution: 0.5%–1% dilution

Warning: Possible drug interactions (check prescriptions). Mucous membrane irritant

Actions: Full-spectrum antimicrobial (diffuse into sick room to reduce airborne microbes)

Primary Compounds: Thymol; phenol

CM Nature: Hot, drying, up

Conditions: Bacterial infections, bronchitis, common cold, cystitis (urinary tract infection), diarrhea, fungal infections, nocturnal enuresis (bedwetting) due to infection, prostatitis, strep throat, viral infections

---

Vetiver *(Vetiveria zizanoides):* root

Dilution: 5%–15% dilution

Warning: None known

Actions: Tonic to the glands of the endocrine, circulatory tonic, emmenagogue

Primary Compounds: Khusimol; sesqiterpenol

CM Nature: Cool, moist, down

Conditions: Bipolar disorder, insomnia, trigeminal neuralgia (facial nerve pain), vertigo

Wintergreen *(Gaultheria procumbens):* leaves

Dilution: 1%–2% dilution

Warning: Possible drug interactions (check prescriptions). Avoid with bleeding disorders. Avoid with salicylate allergies

Actions: Antispasmodic, vasodilatory, anti-inflammatory, pain reducer

Primary Compounds: Methyl salicylate; ester

CM Nature: Warming, drying, up

Conditions: Headaches, pain of all kinds, torticollis (neck spasm, stiff neck)

Yarrow *(Achillea millefolium):* aerial parts

Dilution: 5% dilution

Warning: Possible drug interactions (check prescriptions)

Actions: Choleretic, anti-inflammatory, cicatrisant, styptic

Primary Compounds: Sabinene; monoterpene

CM Nature: Cool, drying, circulating

Conditions: Aphthous ulcers (mouth sores)

Ylang ylang *(Cananga odorata):* flowers

Dilution: 0.5% dilution

Warning: May cause sensitization.

Actions: Antiparasitic, antispasmodic, anti-inflammatory, aphrodisiac

Primary Compounds: α-farnesene; sesquiterpene

CM Nature: Cooling, moisturizing, up

Conditions: Torticollis (neck spasm, stiff neck)

24 Most Useful Essential Oils

1. Black pepper
2. German, or blue, chamomile
3. Roman chamomile
4. Clary sage
5. Clove
6. Cypress
7. Eucalyptus globulus
8. Eucalyptus radiata
9. Fennel
10. Frankincense
11. Geranium
12. Ginger
13. Grapefruit
14. Helichrysum
15. Lavender
16. Oregano
17. Peppermint
18. Ravintsara
19. Rose otto
20. Rosemary
21. Spikenard
22. Tea tree
23. Thyme
24. Vetiver

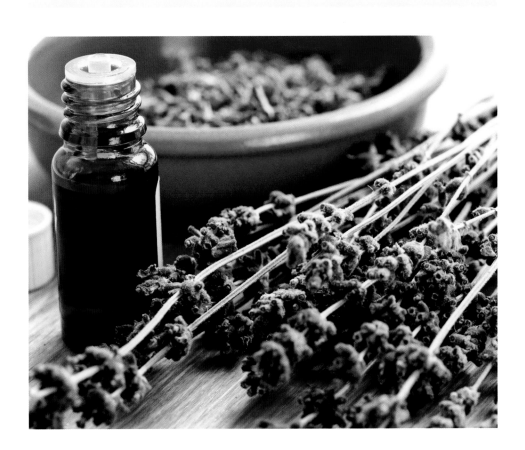

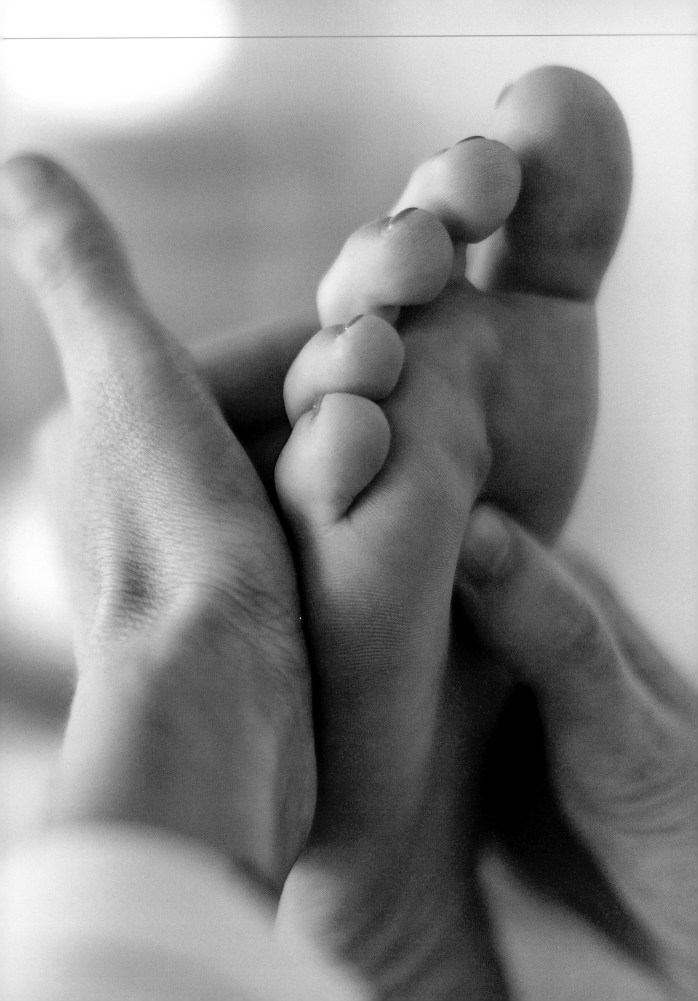

CHAPTER 4

Acupressure and Aromatherapy for Conditions

Effective Techniques for 64 Common Health Conditions

In this chapter, you will find 64 common health conditions that have been chosen because their symptoms may be effectively reduced by acupressure and aromatherapy. Reducing symptoms for any condition can make the recovery process much easier. Even better, these techniques are quite easy to perform on oneself, in the comfort of one's own space.

As described in the Chinese Medicine chapter (see page 8), acupressure is based on the centuries-old practice of acupuncture. Acupuncture uses acupressure points (acupoints) that are mapped out on the body to interact with the flow of qi (energy, or life force) in the patient. Typically, this is done by inserting extremely fine needles at the acupoint, but in the technique described in this book, the treatment is done through pressure and the application of essential oils on each point, both of which are excellent at moving qi. Since most imbalances in the body can be traced to disruptions in the flow of qi, such techniques can be very helpful.

In addition to moving qi, from a Western scientific perspective, essential oils primarily interact with the endocrine and nervous systems. This means that while the treatments work to reduce symptoms, they can also increase a sense of calm and relaxation. The two perspectives — Chinese Medicine and the Western approach — are not mutually exclusive, of course — endocrine changes may explain why the qi is moving, or vice versa. Because stress is at the root of many conditions, these wonderful "side effects" of the treatment really contribute to overall health.

How to Use These Techniques

To use this book effectively, first find the health condition you would like to address, listed here alphabetically under categories that reflect the body's various systems. In addition to a synopsis of the condition, there are suggestions for acupressure points (acupoints) that might help. It is important to be very clear about the point location — directions for locations are found in the "Acupressure Points" chapter, starting on page 18. Also review the directions for applying pressure and time found on pages 21 and 23.

Finally, review the suggested aromatherapy for each acupoint — this section lists those essential oils that are recommended for each condition, which can be added to the treatment to make it more effective. While acupressure and aromatherapy are effective in addressing symptoms, "other treatments" noted here may add an additional support in the treatments of these health conditions.

Proper Dilution

It is very important to use the correct dilution — these can be found, along with other important information about the essential oils, in the chart on page 109.

Reproductive Conditions
Women's Health

Men's Health

Integumentary Conditions (Skin Disorders)

Musculoskeletal Conditions

Endocrine Conditions

Addiction

Addiction is a label used for the condition of being or feeling dependent on a substance, idea, thing or activity. The etiology may be physical, psychological or ideological. Chemical changes in the body may lead to feelings of physical addiction, whereas psychological and ideological addictions often arise from a need for connection.

Many aspects of modern society are difficult to navigate. Feelings of helplessness or lack of power often lead to a desire to escape. For that reason, some people turn to substances that help them feel they can escape situations where they feel trapped.

Signs and Symptoms

Addiction is seen when there is an unmitigated craving for a substance, idea, thing or activity, often to the exclusion of all other aspects of life. Often there are physical and personality changes as the addictive agent takes over the life of the person with an addiction.

Once a person is addicted, there are many behavioral changes. Addicts, for example, often go to extreme measures to ensure they will be able to sustain their habit. Lying, stealing and other radical personality changes are common. With some addiction, there are physical changes as well; in extreme cases, weight loss and fluctuations in energy levels are two common signs, but there may be rapid aging, deterioration of teeth and musculature, and skin ulcers.

Addiction is a very serious condition with potentially grave consequences.

Aromatherapy for Acupoints

Addiction to nicotine: helichrysum on PC6 and LU1

Using drugs to escape reality: vetiver on PC6 and KI1

Addiction to alcohol: angelica on PC6 and LR2

Nervous eating: tangerine or grapefruit on PC6 and SP6

Mental addictions: holy basil on PC6 and Ht7

Note

This section is devoted to helping people with an addiction handle cravings and reduce the need for the addictive agent. Any self-help should be practiced in conjunction with other resources, as addictions are notoriously hard to conquer alone.

Other Treatments

- If any of the aromatherapy suggestions are used on the acupoints, it is a good idea to carry a small vial of the same oil. Sniffing the oil may help reduce cravings
- Vitamin C: intake of vitamin C may help reduce cravings in addicts
- Evening primrose oil may help repair damage that results from addiction

Best Acupressure Point for Addiction

PC6 • Neiguan (see Pericardium 6, page 61)

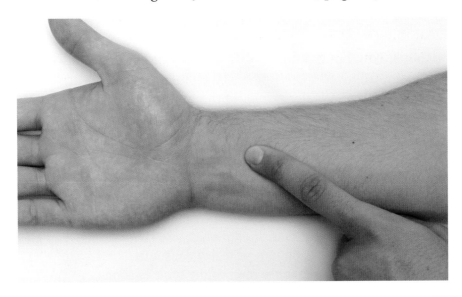

Other Acupressure Points to Consider

After pressing the best acupressure point for this condition, follow with one of these points:

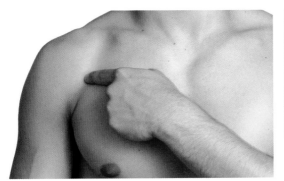

For nicotine addiction, add
LU1 • Zhongfu (see Lung 1, page 24)

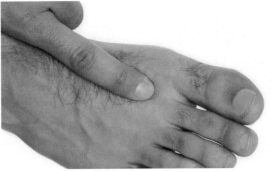

For alcohol addiction, add
LR2 • Xingjian (see Liver 2, page 73)

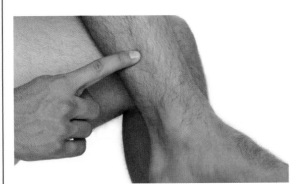

For food addiction, add
SP6 • Sanyinjiao (see Spleen 6, page 43)

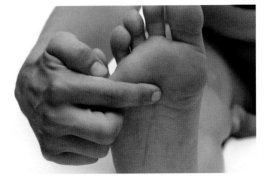

For escapism, add
KI1 • Yongquan (see Kidney 1, page 54)

Adhesive Capsulitis (Frozen Shoulder)

Adhesive capsulitis, commonly known as frozen shoulder, is a condition that causes pain in the shoulder, followed by stiffness. Adhesions form that cause the muscles to stick to each other, dramatically reducing the ability of the muscles to function. The muscle bodies can tear apart with activity, and this tearing leads to the creation of scar tissue, further limiting movement and function.

Frozen shoulder often arises very quickly, in some cases overnight, although it is usually a result of an injury or repetitive movement and poor ergonomics. The after-effects of shoulder surgery (with its associated scar tissue) may develop into adhesive capsulitis, which is why it is so important to exercise the healing joint as soon as comfortably possible. Frozen shoulder will often self-resolve after a period of time; the average healing time is 9 to 18 months.

Signs and Symptoms

The condition starts with severe pain during the "freezing" stage, which fades after a short time to extreme stiffness and radically reduced range of motion. There is often crepitus ("creaking") in the joint. Muscle weakness, combined with the poor range of motion, can effectively take the affected arm out of commission.

Post-menopausal women are most likely to develop frozen shoulder.

Other Treatments

• Add a warm, moist compress or poultice and heating pad to help with stiffness and pain

---

Pain Blend

This pain blend is used to treat multiple conditions. While it can vary slightly with each patient and condition, here's a standard essential oil blend to use: Combine 3 drops of helichrysum, 1 drop of ginger and 1 drop of black pepper in 1 teaspoon (5 mL) of St. John's wort infused oil.

Aromatherapy for Acupoints

Anterior (front) frozen shoulder:
helichrysum on LI15
With pain: on LU7

Posterior (back) frozen shoulder:
helichrysum on TW14
With pain: pain blend (see box) on SI3
With weakness, heaviness: basil on TW14 or KI7
With cold in the joint: black pepper and rosemary on TW14

Best Acupressure Point for Adhesive Capsulitis

LI15 • Jianyu (see Large Intestine 15, page 32)

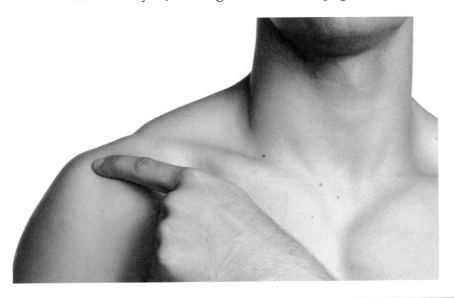

Other Acupressure Points to Consider

After pressing the best acupressure point for this condition, follow with one of these points:

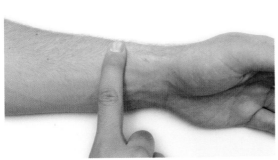

For anterior frozen shoulder with pain, add
LU7 • Lieque (see Lung 7, page 25)

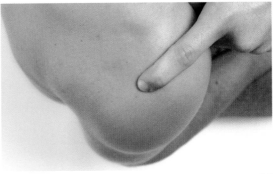

For posterior frozen shoulder with pain, add
TW14 • Jianliao (see Triple Warmer 14,
page 64)

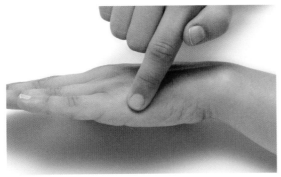

For posterior frozen shoulder with pain, add
SI3 • Houxi (see Small Intestine 3, page 48)

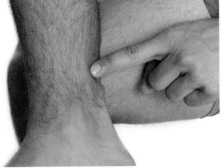

For frozen shoulder accompanied by
weakness and/or heaviness, add
KI7 • Fuliu (see Kidney 7, page 57)

Allergies

Allergies are a hypersensitivity immune response to allergens, defined as substances generally accepted as non-threatening in people without allergies. The immune system mistakes a non-threatening substance as a threat and mounts an exaggerated response. This usually occurs after a period of hypersensitization, where the allergy sufferer has been exposed to the substance over a long time or in large quantities.

Signs and Symptoms

Typical signs and symptoms include itching, sneezing, runny nose, tearing and congestion. Skin allergy signs include redness, rash or hives, itching and blisters.

> ### Note
> This section is designed to help the allergy sufferer reduce their symptoms and is not intended for people suffering from life-threatening reactions such as anaphylaxis.

Other Treatments

- Nettle tea (or capsules) daily for 3 months before the allergy season
- Butterbur capsules may help with respiratory symptoms
- Quercitin, found in onion skins and citrus pith, (or capsules), may help with runny nose, watery eyes and edema due to allergies
- Broth made from onion skins may be taken daily
- Khella capsules may be helpful, especially if there is hay fever, a type of allergy most common when a plant allergen is in bloom

Aromatherapy for Acupoints

Ginger on SP6

Excessive tearing or itchy eyes: chamomile applied very carefully with a cotton bud on BL2

Catarrh (thick mucus and trouble expectorating): inula and eucalyptus on LU7

Wheezing: Hyssopus var. decumbens (not *Hyssopus officinalis*) on LU1

Caution

Hyssopus var. decumbens is not the same as *Hyssopus offinialis*. Be sure to only use Hyssopus var. decumbens essential oil on the recommended acupoint.

Best Acupressure Point for Allergies

SP6 • Sanyinjiao (see Spleen 6, page 43)

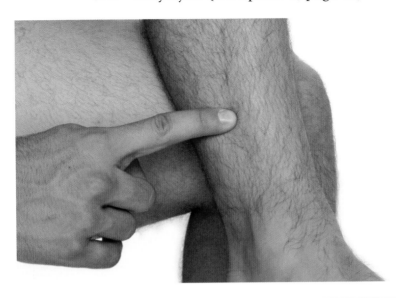

Other Acupressure Points to Consider

After pressing the best acupressure point for this condition, follow with one of these points:

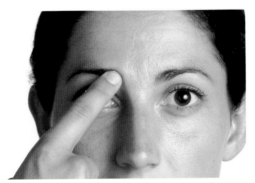

For allergies with watering eyes, add
BL2 • Zanzhu (see Bladder 2, page 50)

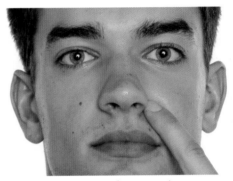

For allergies with excessive watery
mucus, add LI20 • Yingxiang
(see Large Intestine 20, page 33)

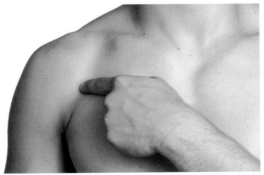

For allergies with wheezing, add
LU1 • Zhongfu (see Lung 1, page 24)

Alopecia (Hair Loss)

There are different types of alopecia, or hair loss, the most common being alopecia areata, or spot baldness. The head and beard are areas that commonly develop alopecia areata, but it can occur anywhere on the body. Alopecia universalis, as it sounds, refers to total hair loss, including eyebrows and eyelashes. In most cases, the follicles remain healthy and the hair will often return with treatment or time.

Most medical experts agree the condition is likely an autoimmune reaction. The inflammation affects the hair follicle so it is unable to function. Most autoimmune disorders are connected to stress in one way or another. The role of stress in alopecia has been studied and a connection established: studies show that most patients initially developed alopecia after a stressful event, and continued stress aggravated the condition.

Signs and Symptoms

Hair loss is the main and often only symptom. There may be irritation or itching at the site.

It has been shown that if more than half the hair falls out in the first occurrence of alopecia, it is more likely to recur, with another flare-up in the future.

While alopecia is not life-threatening, it often occurs with other, more serious conditions. Specifically, it is seen with atopic dermatitis, thyroid disease and diabetes, among other ailments.

Other Treatments

• Figs have been shown to help, so consider adding them to your diet

Aromatherapy for Acupoints

Rosemary on any of the recommended acupressure points, followed by massage

> ## Case Study
>
> Full body massage and scalp treatments can both help reduce stress. It has been found that a topical massage of rosemary verbenone and spike lavender, an essential oil with a camphor content, diluted in a base oil, can both reduce the stress that may lead to alopecia and help stimulate hair growth.

Best Acupressure Point for Alopecia

ST8 • Touwei (see Stomach 8, page 36)

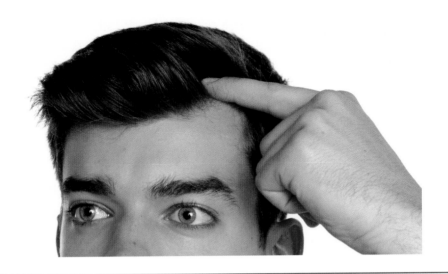

Other Acupressure Points to Consider

After pressing the best acupressure point for this condition, follow with one of these points:

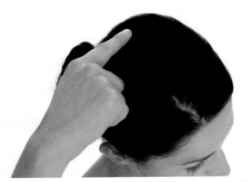

For alopecia at the top of the head, add GV20 • Baihui (see Governing Vessel 20, page 84)

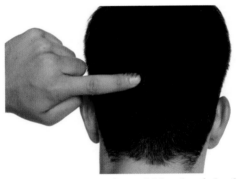

For alopecia at the mid back of the head, add BL9 • Yuzhen (see Bladder 9, page 51)

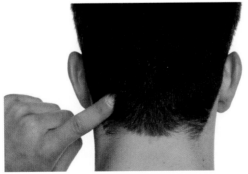

For alopecia on the sides or back of the head, add GB20 • Fengchi (see Gallbladder 20, page 69)

Angina Pectoris (Chest Pain)

Angina pectoris is the medical term for chest pain. Changes in any part of the heart, such as the pericardium, vessels, valves or muscle tissue, may result in pain. It may be accompanied by inflammatory infections of the heart such as rheumatic fever or scarlet fever, although sometimes angina is the after-effect of these conditions. It can be a symptom of a bigger problem, too. Atherosclerosis (coronary artery disease) in particular is the most common cause, but any restriction of blood flow could in theory lead to angina.

Signs and Symptoms

The main symptom of angina is the same as its description — pain felt in the chest. It can manifest primarily as pressure or squeezing with some pain in the jaw, shoulder or arm and is often mistaken for a heart attack, especially in women. The pain can feel shooting or stabbing, burning, dull or aching. Exercise, emotions or stress can all bring on angina pectoris.

> ## Note
> It is important to investigate heart health because angina is a primary symptom of heart disease. If episodes increase in occurrence it may be a situation that needs immediate medical attention — contact a doctor.

Other Treatments

- Hawthorn berry solid extract or caps, linden and motherwort tea, artichoke capsules, guggulipids supplements, CoQ10 supplements, fish oils, niacin and cayenne capsules have been shown to help in various ways
- Dietary changes: eating a fresh, locally grown, whole-foods diet can radically improve heart health

Aromatherapy for Acupoints

Upon exercise (an increase of oxygen): rosemary on PC6 and LU1

With cold and weakness: ginger or rosemary on PC6 and ST36

Stabbing pain: helichrysum on PC6 and LR3; cypress on PC6 and ST40

Burning pain: rose on PC6 and SI1

Best Acupressure Point for Angina Pectoris

PC6 • Neiguan (see Pericardium 6, page 61)

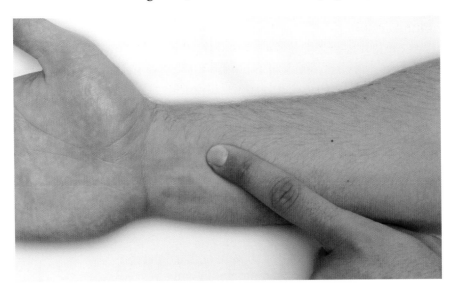

Other Acupressure Points to Consider

After pressing the best acupressure point for this condition, follow with one of these points:

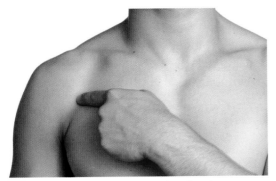

For chest pain upon exercise (an increase of oxygen), add LU1 • Zhongfu (see Lung 1, page 24)

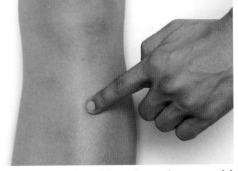

For chest pain with cold and weakness, add ST36 • Zusanli (see Stomach 36, page 39)

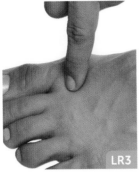

For stabbing chest pain, add LR3 • Taichong (see Liver 3, page 74) or ST40 • Fenglong (see Stomach 40, page 40)

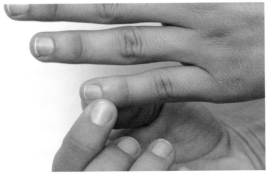

For burning chest pain, add SI1 • Shaoze (see Small Intestine 1, page 47)

Anxiety Disorder

Anxiety disorder occurs when anxiety starts to interrupt normal behavior. While conventional medicine describes anxiety as a serious mental disorder, the symptoms usually occur at all levels of being — mental, emotional, physical and spiritual. It may be felt in the body as physical tension, although most sufferers report the mental restlessness as the most distressing symptom.

In Chinese Medicine, anxiety is seen as a deficiency of trust in the Dao, or the "way" one's life is unfolding. The inability to feel trust may lead to debilitating uncertainty, creating difficulty with decision making.

Signs and Symptoms

There are many different types of anxiety disorders. Each person may manifest a totally different set of symptoms. In general, a person with any type will have increased cortisol levels, the body's typical response to stress. There may be increased sweating, agitated movement and signs of panic. Or the opposite signs may appear — retreat, silence and stillness. Either weight loss or weight gain may be seen.

Anxiety can lead to panic attacks, a greatly heightened emotional response that can cause paralyzing fear and erratic behavior, and physical responses such as tachycardia and palpitations. Some anxiety disorders may lead to a withdrawal from activities of daily living, often due to fear of the panic attack itself, which can occur spontaneously with no apparent trigger when the sufferer is outside of their comfort zone. Agoraphobia may arise as well.

Note
Both hyperthyroidism and adrenal tumor may cause anxiety.

Treating Phobias

For a phobia — a very specific and unreasonable or excessive fear or anxiety associated with a particular trigger — use a calming blend. It will bring calm during anxiety and reprogram the emotional pattern. Find an essential oil or blend that feels calming to you and sniff it at least a few times every day during periods of calm. Consider flower essences — these little treasures have a great track record in helping with emotional imbalances.

Aromatherapy for Acupoints

Rose, lavender on PC6

Lemon balm on Yintang

Spikenard on KI1

Social anxiety: rose on Ht7

Spiritual angst: frankincense and sandalwood on KI9

Pine essential oil represents both down (rooted) and up (pine grows like an arrow to the sky), and can lead to feeling more physically stable

Best Acupressure Point for Anxiety Disorder

PC6 • Neiguan (see Pericardium 6, page 61)

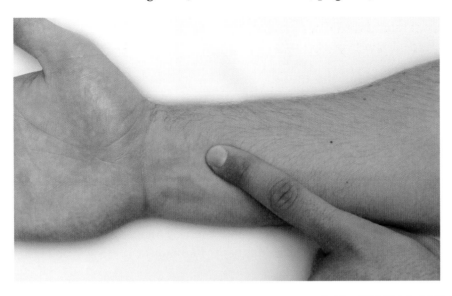

Other Acupressure Points to Consider

After pressing the best acupressure point for this condition, follow with one of these points:

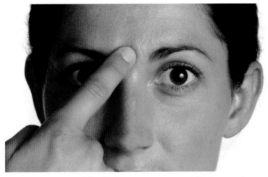

For unspecified (or non-specific) anxiety, add Yintang (see page 87)

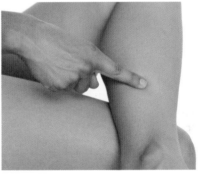

For anxiety due to bipolar disorder, add KI9 • Zhubin (see Kidney 9, page 58)

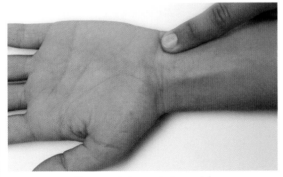

For social anxiety, add Ht7 • Shenmen (see Heart 7, page 46)

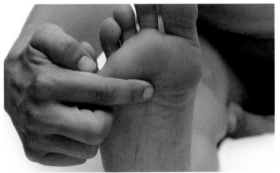

For anxiety that leads to feeling ungrounded, add KI1 • Yongquan (see Kidney 1, page 54)

Aphthous Ulcers (Mouth Sores), Bleeding Gums

Aphthous ulcers (mouth sores) and bleeding gums are both signs of weakened tissues or blood vessels in the mouth. In the case of mouth ulcers, the tissue is irritated and eroded. Bleeding gums indicate weak blood vessels that easily rupture.

Nutritional deficiencies, such as vitamin C and vitamin K, genetic predisposition, drugs (blood thinners) like aspirin; some herbs, such as ginkgo; age, gum disease, gingivitis and pregnancy are all contributing factors. Smoking aggravates both conditions. Aphthous ulcers are understood as indicating excess heat in Chinese Medicine. Bleeding gums are more commonly a condition of yin deficiency.

Signs and Symptoms

Aphthous ulcers are painful and sensitive to the slightest stimulation. Even drinking water can result in pain at the site of the ulcers. Acidic foods are usually intolerable — if the acid gets in the ulcer, the pain is excruciating. Tooth brushing or flossing, occasionally even eating certain foods, can lead to bleeding.

Note
Long-term symptoms may be a sign of a more serious underlying blood imbalance or condition. If the symptoms do not improve or get worse, see a doctor.

Other Treatments
- Mandarin, clove and basil essential oils can all help with mouth pain
- A good calcium/magnesium supplement may help prevent the condition
- A mouth rinse made with goldenseal and myrrh or bee propolis can help to strengthen the gums
- Spilanthes tincture can also strengthen the gums
- The Ayurvedic technique of oil pulling (see box) may help with both conditions

Ayurvedic Oil Pulling
Place a teaspoon of raw sesame oil (with or without the addition of suggested essential oils) into the mouth and swish — attempt to get the oil between all the teeth if possible. Work up to swishing for 20 minutes. Do not swallow!

Aromatherapy for Acupoints

Mouth sores: bay laurel in rose hip seed oil on CV23

Bleeding gums: yarrow or blue chamomile on LI20 if it is mostly in the upper gums, or on ST6 if the bleeding is mostly in the lower gums

Caution
Never use more than one drop at a time when using the mandarin, clove or basil essential oil, and add to a base of aloe vera or sesame oil to swish.

Best Acupressure Point for Aphthous Ulcers and Bleeding Gums

CV23 • Lianquan (see Conception Vessel 23, page 83)

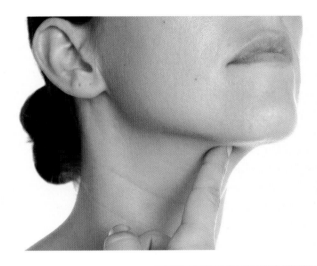

Other Acupressure Points to Consider

After pressing the best acupressure point for this condition, follow with one of these points:

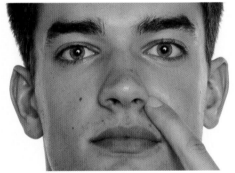

For mostly upper gums, add
LI20 • Yingxiang (see Large Intestine 20, page 33)

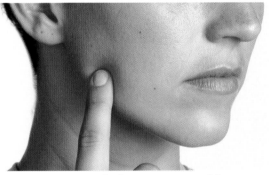

For mostly lower gums, add
ST6 • Jiache (see Stomach 6, page 34)

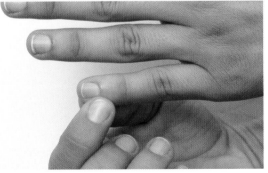

For mouth sores, add
SI1 • Shaoze (see Small Intestine 1, page 47)

Arthritis

Arthritis is a degenerative condition of the joints. Many different kinds of arthritis, including conditions like gout, fall into this category.

Osteoarthritis is usually a result of wear and tear and is more commonly found in people over 60. If the condition develops in a younger person, it usually has a specific etiology, such as injury. The symptoms usually develop and worsen over time. The joint tissues responsible for articulation — namely, the tendons, cartilage and bursae — deteriorate until the bone is no longer cushioned but is working against bone.

Rheumatoid arthritis is an inflammatory autoimmune condition that results in hot, swollen joints. Over time, these inflammatory flares lead to structural changes. As in almost all autoimmune conditions, the symptoms may arise rapidly, a key feature when differentiating this condition from osteoarthritis.

Signs and Symptoms

Osteoarthritis is characterized by increased stiffness and pain and decreased range of motion. As the condition progresses, the connective tissue loses function and atrophies, while the bones enlarge, causing the joints to deform. Women are more likely to develop this condition than men.

Rheumatoid arthritis, like most autoimmune diseases, has flare and remission stages, especially at onset. The longer the inflammatory flares occur, the more permanent damage the joints sustain. Eventually, rheumatoid arthritis results in extreme changes to the joints. In the fingers, a common area to show signs of the disease, the typical change is lateral deviation, so that all the ends of the fingers bend away from the body.

> ## Note
> Arthritis with an acute onset may indicate an infectious process like Lyme disease or a gonococcal infection.

Other Treatments

- Beneficial supplements include glucosamine/chondroitin/MSM, omega-3 fatty acids, calcium/magnesium, devil's claw, ginger, turmeric and boswellia (especially for rheumatoid)

Aromatherapy for Acupoints

Osteoarthritis of the upper body: Roman chamomile on SI3

Osteoarthritis of the lower body, especially knees: juniper berry on BL40

Rheumatoid arthritis in joints of the upper body: eucalyptus citriodora on SI1

Rheumatoid arthritis of the lower body: eucalyptus citriodora on GB34

Stiffness and pain: pain blend (see page 136) on GB34

Best Acupressure Point for Arthritis

SI3 • Houxi (see Small Intestine 3, page 48)

Also recommended for: osteoarthritis of the upper body

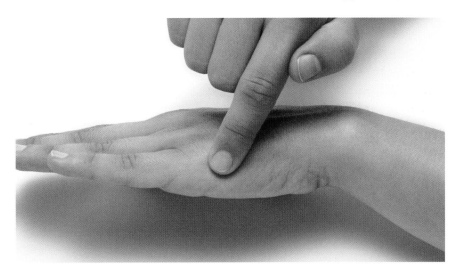

Other Acupressure Points to Consider

After pressing the best acupressure point for this condition, follow with one of these points:

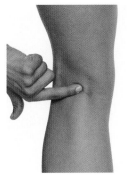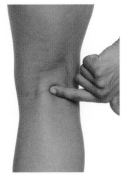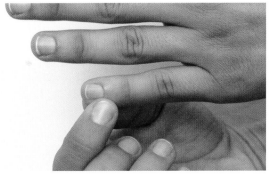

For osteoarthritis of the lower body, especially knees, add BL40 • Weizhong (see Bladder 40, page 52)

For rheumatoid arthritis in joints of the upper body, add SI1 • Shaoze (see Small Intestine 1, page 47)

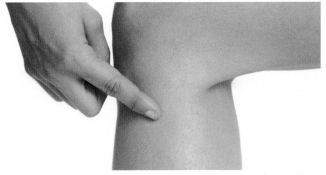

For rheumatoid arthritis of the lower body, or for stiffness and pain from rheumatoid arthritis or osteoarthritis, add GB34 • Yanglingquan (see Gallbladder 34, page 71)

Asthma

Asthma is really best understood by an alternative name — reactive airway disease. The sufferer experiences a decrease in available air as the bronchial tubes narrow in response to a trigger, such as an allergen or environmental pollutant. The bronchial tubes constrict and increase the production of thick, sticky secretions in an attempt to protect the lungs from the trigger. Until recently, non-allergic asthma was not considered an autoimmune disease, but recent studies have led to a reevaluation of the disease.

Signs and Symptoms

Symptoms include productive or dry cough, wheezing, shortness of breath, gasping, inability to converse normally and possibly cyanosis (a bluish discoloration of the skin resulting from inadequate oxygenation of the blood). A person experiencing an asthma attack often adopts the tripod position in an attempt to use accessory muscles to help the lungs receive a greater air supply. Typically this posture involves being seated but bending forward, hands on knees, which allows the individual to engage the muscles of the neck, shoulders and chest.

Note

While regularly treating the points may help reduce the incidence of asthma attacks, these treatments are *not advised for acute attacks*. The condition known as status asthmaticus is a life-threatening variant that can escalate rapidly into respiratory failure. Do not hesitate to seek medical attention if symptoms of asthma arise.

Other Treatments

- Khella caps, B_6 and B_{12}, magnesium, borage or black currant seed oil caps can be helpful
- Warm (not hot!) steam inhalations of the essential oils listed above
- Apply a warm compress on the chest, or add to a foot bath for severely sensitive people
- Consider pain blend (see page 136) on exhausted accessory muscles after the asthma attack has resolved

Aromatherapy for Acupoints

For children: Roman chamomile, frankincense on LU1, KI26

For adults: Hyssopus var. decumbens (not *Hyssopus officinalis*) on KI3

Asthma due to anxiety: rosemary on KI27

Asthma due to an upper respiratory condition: cypress on LU11

Caution

When considering essential oils for any breathing disorder, it is imperative to proceed with great caution. Please review the directions for introducing essential oils in a safe manner (page 105).

Best Acupressure Point for Asthma

Dingchuan (see page 86)

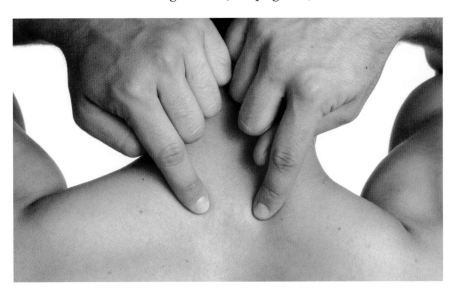

Other Acupressure Points to Consider

After pressing the best acupressure point for this condition, follow with one of these points:

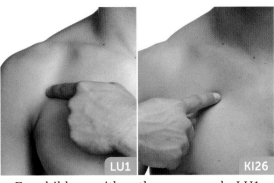

For children with asthma, use only LU1
• Zhongfu (see Lung 1, page 24), KI26 •
Yuzhong (see Kidney 26, page 59)

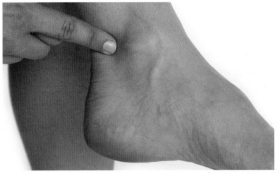

For adults with asthma, add
KI3 • Taixi (see Kidney 3, page 55)

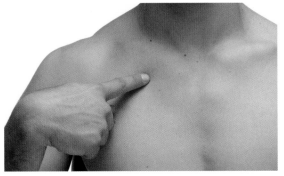

For asthma due to anxiety, add
KI27 • Shufu (see Kidney 27, page 60)

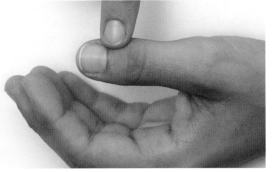

For asthma due to an upper respiratory
condition, add LU11 • Shaoshang
(see Lung 11, page 28)

Atopic Dermatitis (Eczema)

Atopic dermatitis (eczema) is an inflammatory condition of the skin. The latest findings suggest it is an autoimmune condition. Two proteins have been determined to act as antigens, and drugs blocking the signalling of these proteins have been found to reduce symptoms.

The hygiene hypothesis suggests that children raised in hyper-sterilized homes are more likely to develop both eczema and asthma, two conditions commonly seen together. When a child encounters a trigger, a flare-up occurs. Unfortunately, nearly anything can act as a trigger, but more recently the main culprits have been soap, shampoo, detergents and synthetic and chemical additives in topical skin-care products. Baby eczema is very common — switching laundry detergent to something more natural and gentle often resolves the issue.

Signs and Symptoms

Each case of eczema is distinctive in presentation, but generally there will be an itchy red raised rash. Tiny blisters often appear; as they develop they may ooze, a development that frequently leads to cracked skin. If the condition continues, the cracks may bleed and scab. The hardened tissue then easily reopens, making it difficult to heal.

Note

Excessive use of topical steroids for eczema is believed to drive the condition deeper into the system, often manifesting later as asthma. Avoid topical steroids if at all possible.

Homemade Repair Salve

Treat eczema at night by applying a repair salve, easily made at home. The recipe is found on page 170 (see Chest Rub box) but make these modifications to it: Use 2 oz caulophyllum oil for the base instead of coconut oil. Add up to 30 drops of essential oils — consider eucalyptus citriodora or lemongrass, helichrysum and lavender. Bee propolis, myrrh powder or benzoin may also be added. (*Caution:* bee products may cause allergies in some people.)

Aromatherapy for Acupoints

Eucalyptus citriodora or lemongrass on LI11

Red, hot skin: blue chamomile and helichrysum on LU7

Dry, cracked, bleeding eczema: German chamomile on SP10

With asthma: frankincense on SP6

Best Acupressure Point for Atopic Dermatitis

LI11 • Quchi (see Large Intestine 11, page 31)

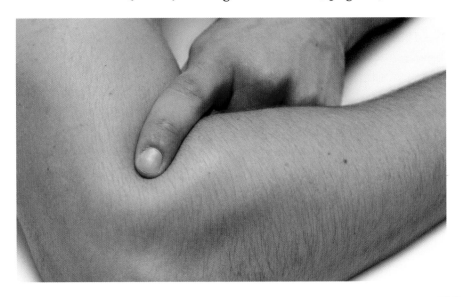

Other Acupressure Points to Consider

After pressing the best acupressure point for this condition, follow with one of these points:

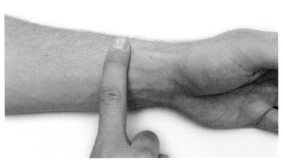

For atopic dermatitis with red, hot skin, add
LU7 • Lieque (see Lung 7, page 25)

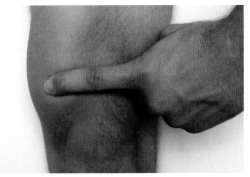

For dry, cracked, bleeding eczema, add
SP10 • Xuehai (see Spleen 10, page 45)

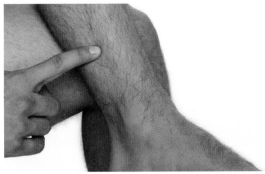

For atopic dermatitis concurrent with
asthma, add SP6 • Sanyinjiao
(see Spleen 6, page 43)

Bacterial Infections

These infections are caused by bacteria and can occur in any system anywhere in the body. Some bacterial infections are easily addressed, while others can be fatal.

Signs and Symptoms

Symptoms include heat, redness and pain at the site of infection. If the area is open, there may be discharge to the surface; for example, bacterial infections of the eye will lead to purulent discharge (pus) and tearing as the body clears the bacteria and white blood cells that have been destroyed in the healing process. If the condition is internal, the more overt signs are fever and pain. If the infection spreads or worsens, a sweet smell may exude from the pores.

Staphylococcus aureus is a bacterium that occurs naturally on the human body but in certain situations can become life-threatening very quickly. As patients with decreased immune function are treated in an overly sanitized hospital environment, they are at risk of contracting necrotizing fasciitis, commonly called flesh-eating disease, an infection that rapidly destroys deep layers of tissue. The radical sterilization measures required in the hospital setting have resulted in bacteria able to resist the strongest antibiotics available. Even if the disease is not fatal, a patient can be left disfigured.

Note
All bacterial infections should be diagnosed by a physician, as some may worsen rapidly and become extremely serious.

Other Treatments
- Vitamin C, echinacea and garlic
- Lemon juice diluted in warm water for hydration
- Apple cider vinegar wash (see box, right)

Aromatherapy for Acupoints

Thyme or oregano on LI4

With heat: lavender on LI11

Respiratory involvement: thyme or cypress on LU7

With fatigue: black spruce on SP6

Apple Cider Vinegar Wash

To make a wash to treat bacterial infections, add 2 tablespoons (30 mL) of apple cider vinegar to 8 ounces (250 mL) water.

Essential Oils and Infection

Nearly all EOs are antibacterial, although some are very potent and more specific. Any EO high in phenolic compounds like thymol and carvacrol are very active against bacteria. They are also extremely potent and can damage tissue if not used carefully. One drop diluted in 1 teaspoon (5 mL) of base oil (1% dilution) is effective and safe, but definitely plan to do a patch test first (see page 105).

Another option is to use the fresh herb. When a larger area of tissue is threatened with infection, a wash made from thyme and oregano may be more effective. Steep the herbs in hot water, then the steeped herbs may be applied directly to the wound as an herb pack (wrap the herbs in muslin first). Garlic was traditionally added to this formula, so it may be added if desired.

Best Acupressure Point for Bacterial Infections

LI4 • Hegu (see Large Intestine 4, page 29)

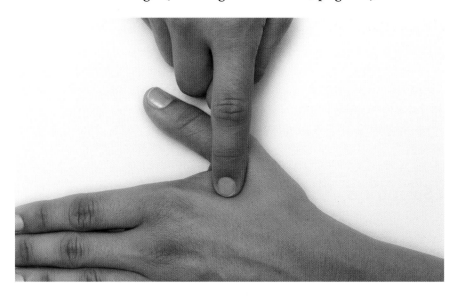

Other Acupressure Points to Consider

After pressing the best acupressure point for this condition, follow with one of these points:

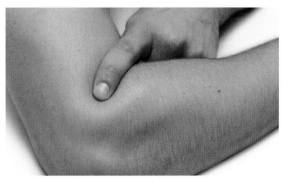

For bacterial infections with heat, add
LI11 • Quchi (see Large Intestine 11,
page 31)

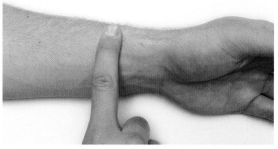

For bacterial infections with respiratory
involvement, add LU7 • Lieque
(see Lung 7, page 25)

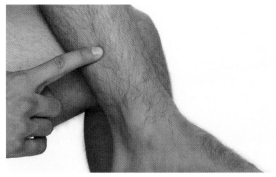

For bacterial infections with fatigue, add
SP6 • Sanyinjiao (see Spleen 6, page 43)

Bipolar Disorder

Bipolar disorder is characterized by states that vacillate between mania and depression. There are several categories of the condition, depending on how it manifests: it may be a short-term situation or a lifelong struggle. The cause of this disorder is unknown, but research suggests a genetic link. If there is a history of the disease in the immediate family, it is more likely to develop. Certainly neurotransmitter imbalances play a role. Both emotional and physiological trauma have been implicated as well.

Signs and Symptoms

Mania usually manifests as great energy and enthusiasm and a reduced need for sleep or rest, and is often marked by extreme creativity. Some experience hallucinations or delusions. Manic patients usually experience this extreme until their physical resources wear out, at which point they fall into depression, characterized by exhaustion, lack of energy for activities of daily living and no inclination to engage with society and life in general. Bipolar disorder exhibits both depression and mania, so if either state manifests without the other, it is a different disorder.

Erratic and dangerous behavior is often seen in the manic phase. Patients often cannot see or are unwilling to accept limitations — they may even believe they are superhuman. Meanwhile, many patients are considered suicide risks in the depressive phase.

> ### Note
> The suggestions provided here are designed to reduce the likelihood of a major event and mostly aim to achieve balance. If events attributed to the disorder are causing disruptions to everyday life, a doctor should be consulted.

Other Treatments

• Lemon balm (melissa) makes a wonderful tea to help maintain balance. To make your own tea, place a small handful of fresh lemon balm leaves in a teapot and steep, covered, for 5 minutes before drinking

Accessing Resources for Bipolar Disorder

Many resources are available to help patients with bipolar disorder. The difficult part, however, lies in seeking such help. Patients in the manic phase believe they don't need help, and in the depressive phase they don't have the impetus to seek help.

Aromatherapy for Acupoints

Melissa on KI9

Manic phase: frankincense on Ht7, vetiver on KI1

Depressive phase: rose on SP6

With anger: helichrysum on LR2

With euphoria and hallucinations: vetiver on PC6, KI1, GV26

Essential oils are wonderful allies to reprogram responses. If the oil is inhaled regularly in times of relative balance — that is, only when a person is feeling balanced — the same oil may help return the individual to a balanced state if inhaled during extreme mood swings.

Best Acupressure Point for Bipolar Disorder
KI9 • Zhubin (see Kidney 9, page 58)

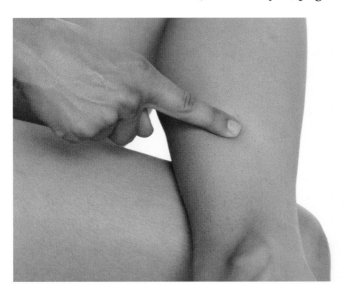

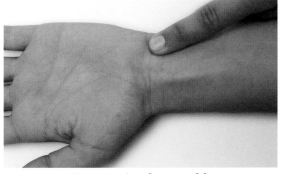

Other Acupressure Points to Consider

After pressing the best acupressure point for this condition, follow with one of these points:

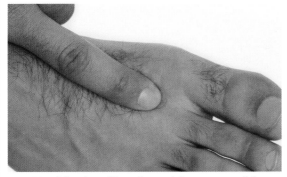

For manic phase, add
Ht7 • Shenmen (see Heart 7, page 46)

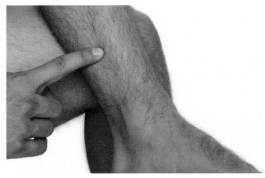

For depressive phase, add
SP6 • Sanyinjiao (see Spleen 6, page 43)

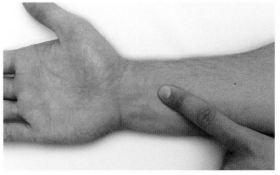

For bipolar disorder with anger, add
LR2 • Xingjian (see Liver 2, page 73)

For bipolar disorder with euphoria
and hallucinations, add PC6 • Neiguan
(see Pericardium 6, page 61)

Bloating

Bloating is typically due to retention of gas in the gastrointestinal tract, but it can also be caused by retained fluids or stool. Bloating may be caused by overeating, eating foods that are difficult to digest, food sensitivities or allergies, constipation or eating while experiencing stress. Many digestive disorders, such as inflammatory bowel disease (IBD) or celiac disease, may also present with bloating. In babies, the condition of bloating is called colic.

Signs and Symptoms

The most common symptom is swelling, but it is often accompanied by discomfort or pain in the gut. There is an increased likelihood of flatulence, especially if food sensitivities are the causative factor. There may be decreased appetite, nausea and vomiting. Irritability is common.

> ### Note
> Intestinal obstruction can result in bloating, and may be an emergency situation. Bloating may also be a symptom of many diseases, including a number of different kinds of cancer and liver disease. If the bloating is from an undiagnosed cause or worsens suddenly, see a doctor.

Other Treatments
- Aniseed, fennel, coriander, cumin and/or cardamom, made into tea or taken in capsule form
- Herbal digestive bitters before meals often help alleviate bloating

Abdominal Massage
Lie on your left side. Starting at the lower right quadrant (near the top of the right hip bone), slowly and gently massage around the abdomen in small circular motions, moving up the right side, across under the ribs and down the left side until the discomfort is relieved. Adding a drop of peppermint essential oil dilution really helps.

Aromatherapy for Acupoints

With pain: fennel on CV12

With nausea: peppermint on PC6

With diarrhea: ginger on ST25

Best Acupressure Point for Bloating
ST36 • Zusanli (see Stomach 36, page 39)

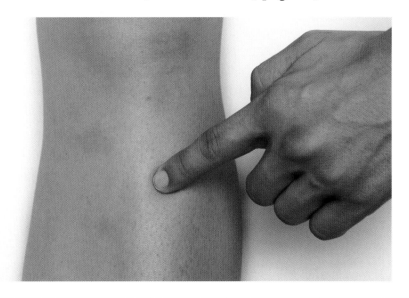

Other Acupressure Points to Consider

After pressing the best acupressure point for this condition, follow with one of these points:

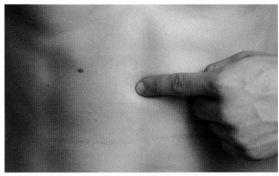

For bloating with pain, add
CV12 • Zhongwan (see Conception
Vessel 12, page 80)

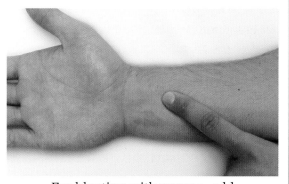

For bloating with nausea, add
PC6 • Neiguan (see Pericardium 6, page 61)

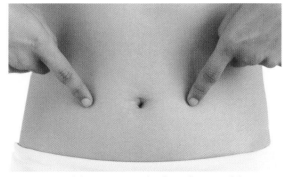

For bloating with diarrhea, add
ST25 • Tianshu (see Stomach 25, page 38)

Bowel Incontinence

With this condition, patients experience a decreased control over bowel movements. It may be temporary, as in the case of food poisoning, when the body's natural defenses are trying to clear toxins as quickly as possible. It may occur as a result of nerve damage following childbirth or surgery, or because of chronic disease, such as diabetes. Increased age also leads to less muscle tone; anal leakage is common in the elderly. Men who have prostate cancer often have a greater likelihood of bowel incontinence, either due to structural change or treatment.

Digestive disorders like ulcerative colitis or irritable bowel disease (IBD) can have bowel incontinence as a symptom.

Signs and Symptoms
Loss of bowel control is the main sign. There may be pain or cramping if it is a result of food poisoning, or it may be accompanied by blood if the cause is a gastrointestinal disorder. If the condition occurs because of age, the leakage may be a small amount, while other causes may result in explosive diarrhea.

Anal leakage is usually a fairly benign result of age, but if the stool is bloody, it may be a sign of a more serious condition. If it is from food poisoning, treat the cause.

Note
If symptoms get worse or if the volume of stool loss goes up dramatically, see a doctor.

Other Treatments
- Witch hazel is an astringent and, applied topically, can help tone lax tissues of the anus
- Add more fiber and healthy oils like flax to the diet; stay hydrated for better stool formation
- Kegel exercises help strengthen the pelvic floor
- Hyaluronic acid capsules may help repair the structures of the anus
- Herbs (in capsules) may also be helpful: boswellia, aloe, peppermint

Reassessing Diet
An elimination diet to uncover possible irritants in the diet may be necessary. Many foods, including meat, red wine and sulfur-containing foods, are known to cause relapses in patients with ulcerative colitis, a leading cause of bowel incontinence.

Aromatherapy for Acupoints

Frankincense on CV1

Due to age: blue chamomile on CV4, KI3

After long illness: basil on SP6

Due to anal prolapse: peppermint on GV20

Best Acupressure Point for Bowel Incontinence

CV1 • Huiyin (see Conception Vessel 1, page 76)

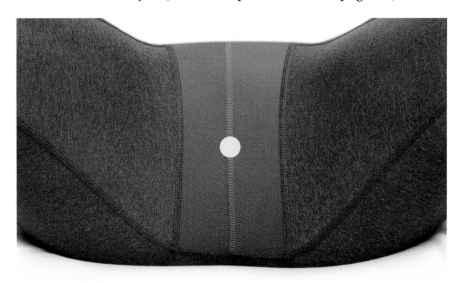

Other Acupressure Points to Consider

After pressing the best acupressure point for this condition, follow with one of these points:

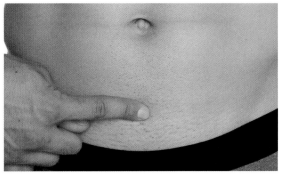

For bowel incontinence due to age, add CV4 • Guanyuan (see Conception Vessel 4, page 78)

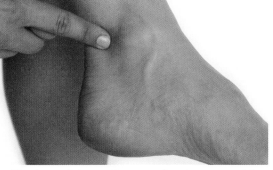

For bowel incontinence due to age, add KI3 • Taixi (see Kidney 3, page 55)

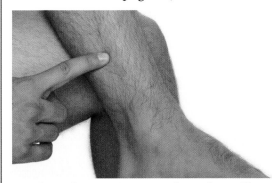

For bowel incontinence after a long illness, add SP6 • Sanyinjiao (see Spleen 6, page 43)

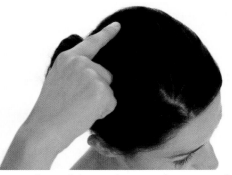

For bowel incontinence due to anal prolapse, add GV20 • Baihui (see Governing Vessel 20, page 84)

Bronchitis

Bronchitis is an inflammatory condition of the bronchial tubes of the respiratory system; specifically, it affects the mucous membrane lining of the bronchioles. Bronchitis can manifest acutely or it may be chronic. With acute bronchitis, the cause is usually a microbial infection — bacteria, viruses and fungi are all possible causes. It can also be an autoimmune condition.

Signs and Symptoms

Inflammation and increased secretions lead to difficulty breathing and shortness of breath. Coughing is common as the lungs attempt to clear the restriction. If it is an acute condition, there are often other symptoms of infection, such as purulent mucus or fever. Chronic bronchitis may result from repeated bouts of the acute version, which damages the tissue. The scarring causes persistent difficulty breathing.

People suffering from bronchitis often adopt the tripod position — seated, bending forward with the hands on the knees — in an attempt to engage accessory muscles of the neck and chest to assist in the breathing process. The posture is usually assumed by those in respiratory distress, as they lose function slowly enough to be unaware of how restricted their breathing has become.

Cigarette smokers often develop chronic bronchitis. Smoking will exacerbate both acute and chronic bronchitis because smoking destroys the cilia responsible for sweeping debris up and out of the lungs.

> ### Note
> Acute bronchitis can rapidly become an emergency situation — if symptoms are severe, do not rely on the protocols described here but contact a doctor.

Other Treatments

- Inula and eucalyptus: as mucolytic agents and expectorants, they help break down and move phlegm
- Inhalation therapy in very warm (not boiling!) water: add a drop of pine or peppermint to help open the air passages (see page 226)
- One drop of thyme in a foot bath, or thyme capsules
- Add more garlic and onions to the diet. If making a broth, make sure to add the papery skins of onions (skins removed before serving) — they are high in quercitin, a substance known to improve respiratory health
- Lobelia tincture is very effective at opening the airways and helping expel phlegm

Aromatherapy for Acupoints

Acute bronchitis: eucalyptus globulus on LU7

Chronic bronchitis: fir on ST36

With sore throat: Ravintsara on CV22

With pain in the chest and heart pain: rose sandalwood on CV17

Caution

Be very careful when considering essential oils for any respiratory condition. Once you have determined an oil to be safe for use (see page 96), apply it to the bottom of the foot first — it is far from the nose and much less likely to cause constriction in the respiratory system.

Best Acupressure Point for Bronchitis
LU7 • Lieque (see Lung 7, page 25)

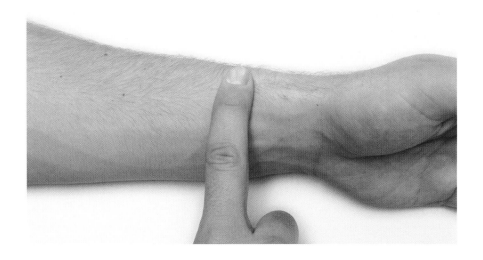

Other Acupressure Points to Consider

After pressing the best acupressure point for this condition, follow with one of these points:

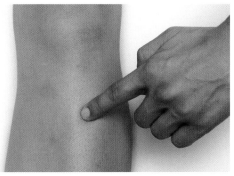

For chronic bronchitis, add
ST36 • Zusanli (see Stomach 36, page 39)

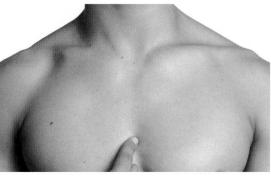

For bronchitis with pain in the chest and heart pain, add CV17 • Tanzhong (see Conception Vessel 17, page 81)

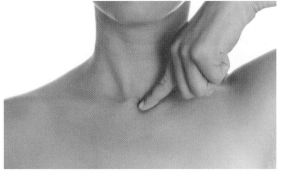

For bronchitis with sore throat, add
CV22 • Tiantu (see Conception Vessel 22, page 82)

Bruising and Hematoma

Bruises occur when an injury leads to ruptured capillaries. The blood that escapes the vessels pools under the skin. Inflammation in the area makes it hard for the leaked blood to be cleared, which leads to a short-term discoloration at the site. A hematoma is a larger area of leaked blood that has clotted at the site. This leads to a raised mound with a slightly gelatinous feel.

Signs and Symptoms

The main sign is redness, followed by a dark blue to black or purple discoloration that eventually changes into green and yellow before fading completely. Some particularly bad bruises may leave a permanent darkening of the tissue. Pain, swelling and irritation usually accompany injuries that lead to bruises.

> ## Note
> A subdural hematoma (occurring under the dura mater of the brain) is a very serious condition that usually requires surgery to relieve the pressure on the brain.

Other Treatments

- Helichrysum in caulophyllum base oil is the best combination to move the stagnant blood of a bruise or hematoma
- Vitamin C, vitamin K, iron, bioflavanoids, quercetin and bromelain may help
- Garlic, fish oil, CoQ10 and ginkgo — all these supplements can help with circulation, but they can also potentially increase the likelihood of bruising

Aromatherapy for Acupoints

Helichrysum on SP10

Frequent bruising: carrot seed on LR3

Due to illness or debility: rose on SP6

Best Acupressure Point for Bruising and Hematoma

SP10 • Xuehai (see Spleen 10, page 45)

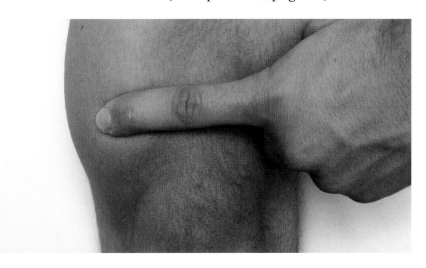

Other Acupressure Points to Consider

After pressing the best acupressure point for this condition, follow with one of these points:

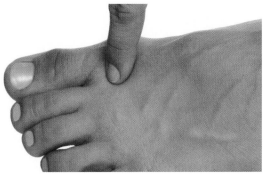 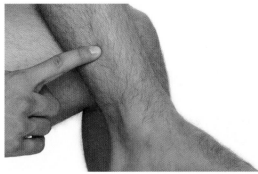

For frequent bruising; for bruising and hematoma with blood disorders, add LR3 • Taichong (see Liver 3, page 74)

For bruising and hematoma due to illness or debility, add SP6 • Sanyinjiao (see Spleen 6, page 43)

Carpal Tunnel Syndrome

The term refers to a collection of symptoms resulting from pressure on the median nerve, the primary nerve serving the hand and fingers. With this condition, the median nerve becomes trapped in the carpal tunnel, a small gap created by the transverse carpal ligament and the bones of the wrist. In addition to the nerve, the tendons responsible for moving the fingers pass through this small space. If inflammation of the tissues occurs as a result of overuse (repetitive movements like typing, for example), the nerve is caught between the swollen tissue and the bones, resulting in diminished function.

The median nerve innervates the thumb, the first and second fingers, and half of the third finger, as well as the nail beds of these fingers. The nerve is also responsible for bringing sensation to the skin of these fingers and some parts of the hand. The lateral (outer) side of the hand and the pinky (fifth) finger are served by a different nerve, and carpal tunnel syndrome is often confirmed by normal sensations in the pinky.

Signs and Symptoms

In addition to diminished function, carpal tunnel syndrome usually results in tingling, numbness and fatigue of the hand. There is often associated pain — often sharp and stabbing — and there may be an electric sensation. Pain may radiate to other areas, commonly up the arm toward the elbow.

Proper ergonomics when performing repetitive tasks is crucial. Many computer keyboards are designed to keep the hands in a more natural position when typing, while pads can help support the wrists.

The condition may spontaneously reverse and normal function return with no treatment whatsoever; however, this is not usual. The conventional treatment is surgery, and braces may be helpful in some cases. Oral corticosteroids are also regularly prescribed.

Note

Carpal tunnel syndrome may be associated with other diseases such as hypothyroidism and diabetes, and pregnancy can exacerbate the condition.

Other Treatments

- Acupuncture: Chinese Medicine has had success in reducing pain and other symptoms using a technique called wet cupping
- Stretches to lengthen the structures involved in the entrapment can be very helpful

Aromatherapy for Acupoints

Frankincense in St. John's wort oil on PC7

With heat: helichrysum on LU11

With cold: pain blend (see page 136) on Ht7

Best Acupressure Point for Carpal Tunnel Syndrome

PC7 • Daling (see Pericardium 7, page 62)

Also recommended for: carpal tunnel syndrome with contracture

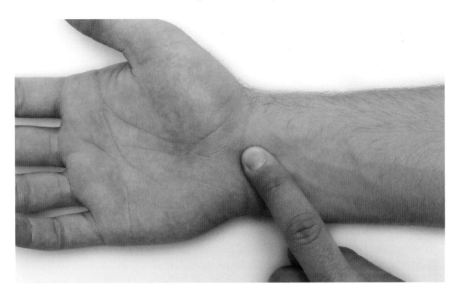

Other Acupressure Points to Consider

After pressing the best acupressure point for this condition, follow with one of these points:

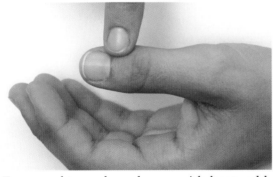

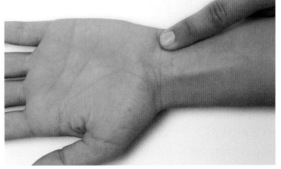

For carpal tunnel syndrome with heat, add LU11 • Shaoshang (see Lung 11, page 28)

For carpal tunnel syndrome with cold, use Ht7 • Shenmen (see Heart 7, page 46)

Chronic Fatigue

Characterized by an unrelenting lack of energy, chronic fatigue is difficult to diagnose since it may accompany most conditions. There are nearly as many causes of fatigue as there are people who suffer from it.

Nutritional deficiencies and malabsorption are commonly the cause. Chronic fatigue syndrome (CFS), the incidence of which is increasing at an alarming rate, is a collection of symptoms that includes fatigue. Exposure to concentrated doses of some substances, especially mercury, mold, pesticides and xenoestrogens from plastics, has been implicated in the onset of condition.

Chronic fatigue may also be linked to adrenal fatigue — a weakening of the HPA (hypothalamic-pituitary-adrenal) axis. When the HPA axis is overstimulated, usually from consistent exposure to stressors, it will function less optimally. With constant overstimulation, the adrenal glands reach a point where they simply cannot react to stimulating hormones anymore: they become unable to react to stress. As the endocrine system is so interdependent, other parts will attempt to take on the role, causing them to fatigue and reducing the system even further.

Signs and Symptoms

The most common symptom is a pervasive sense of feeling unwell, or the sense of what is often referred to as malaise. The body and limbs feel heavier than usual. All activities of daily living become more challenging. Fatigue is often found together with a reduced interest in activities, for obvious reasons, as this symptom can affect all aspects of health, including mental, emotional and physical.

If not addressed, adrenal fatigue can deteriorate into adrenal exhaustion — a much more serious situation requiring rehabilitation.

> ## Note
> If you find yourself with the above signs or symptoms and they are getting worse or not improving, see a doctor. Dizziness and loss of consciousness may be a sign of a more serious condition. Seek medical attention.

Other Treatments

- Sleep when the source of fatigue is overwork
- B vitamins, vitamin D and CoQ10
- Licorice solid extract, or Siberian ginseng solid extract if there is a diagnosis of hypertension, as licorice may increase blood pressure if taken long term

Aromatherapy for Acupoints

Adrenal fatigue: geranium on KI3, black spruce on the lower back, under the lowest ribs, as needed

With sleeplessness: orange and spikenard on KI1, 30 minutes before bed (see Insomnia)

With cold: geranium on SP6 or KI3

Due to debility: ginger on CV4

Sleep Trouble?

Patients report low energy that they cannot replenish, no matter how many hours of sleep or rest they get. The condition may result in more time sleeping or, on the contrary, it may make it more difficult to sleep. Typically, people with CFS or adrenal fatigue do not feel refreshed by sleep.

Best Acupressure Point for Chronic Fatigue

KI3 • Taixi (see Kidney 3, page 55)

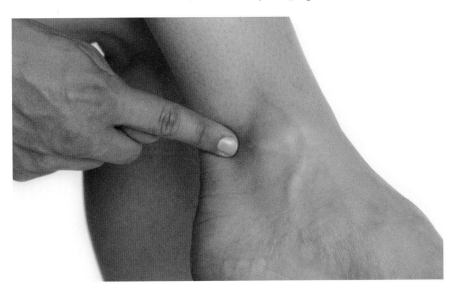

Other Acupressure Points to Consider

After pressing the best acupressure point for this condition, follow with one of these points:

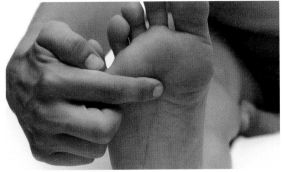

Also add KI1 • Yongquan
(see Kidney 1, page 54)

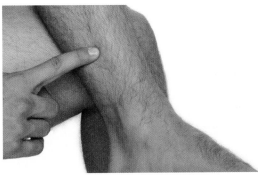

For chronic fatigue with cold, add
SP6 • Sanyinjiao (see Spleen 6, page 43)

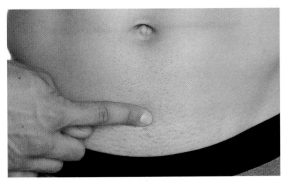

For chronic fatigue due to debility,
add CV4 • Guanyuan
(see Conception Vessel 4, page 78)

Common Cold

The common cold is viral infection resulting in a typical (common) set of symptoms. The main culprits are respiratory syncytial virus, rotovirus, rhinovirus and coronavirus. These viruses can survive on surfaces outside of the body long enough to infect others — most people catch a cold when they come in contact with the causative agent after someone sneezes or coughs. Doorknobs and light switches, for example, are surfaces we regularly touch without thinking.

Those most at risk include babies and children, the elderly and the immunocompromised. If the immune system is weakened or suppressed, a simple common cold can be a serious problem.

Signs and Symptoms
Stiff neck, fatigue, a feeling of general malaise, headache, sore throat, fever and chills, sneezing, coughing, runny nose and other symptoms can manifest with the common cold.

Other Treatments
- One drop Ravintsara essential oil in 1 teaspoon (5 mL) of honey if a sore throat accompanies the cold. Allow to slowly melt in the mouth and trickle down the throat
- Chest rub with thyme linalool, peppermint, eucalyptus and Hyssopus var. decumbens, depending on age or respiratory status (see box)
- A respiratory herbal blend in caps, or a tincture when there is thick catarrh that is difficult to expectorate
- Garlic and onion soup, preferably made with a bone broth base

Chest Rub

Gently melt 1/4 cup (60 mL) of coconut oil and 1 tablespoon (15 mL) of shaved beeswax (beeswax pellets may be used) over low heat. Pour mixture into an empty jar to cool. After it has cooled but before it sets up, stir in 4 drops of thyme linalool, 8 drops of peppermint, 8 drops of eucalyptus, 4 drops of Hyssopus var. decumbens essential oils. Stir well to combine. After patch testing on the foot or elbow, apply to the chest as a rub, massaging in well, as needed. Be sure to introduce this slowly in small amounts.

Aromatherapy for Acupoints

With chills:
For children: eucalyptus radiata on LU7
For adults: cinnamon and eucalyptus globulus on LU7

With fever:
For children: orange and eucalyptus radiata on LI4
For adults: peppermint and eucalyptus globulus on LI4

With fatigue: geranium on SP6

With alternating chills and fever: basil on GB43

Best Acupressure Point for Common Cold
LU7 • Lieque (see Lung 7, page 25)

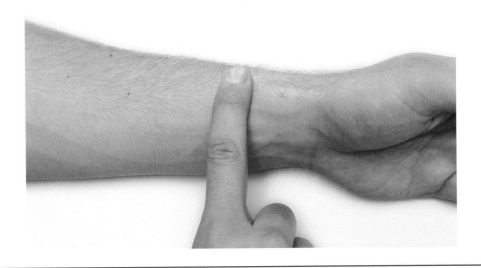

Other Acupressure Points to Consider

After pressing the best acupressure point for this condition, follow with one of these points:

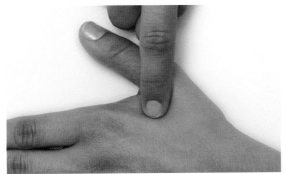

For cold with fever, add
LI4 • Hegu (see Large Intestine 4, page 29)

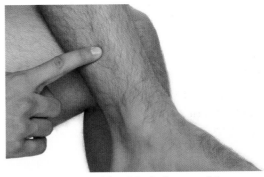

For cold with fatigue, add
SP6 • Sanyinjiao (see Spleen 6, page 43)

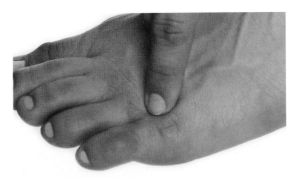

For cold with alternating chills and fever,
add GB43 • Xiaxi (see Gallbladder 43,
page 72)

Conjunctivitis (Pinkeye)

Conjunctivitis is an inflammation of the conjunctiva of the eye. This condition is often referred to by its common name, pinkeye, and may be caused by bacterial or viral agents, or by irritation from pollutants or allergens. Contact lens wearers often develop pinkeye from the lens itself, especially if the lenses are old or degraded.

Signs and Symptoms

Reddening of the conjunctiva, excessive tearing, itching, burning eyes and blurred vision are possible symptoms of the condition. If pinkeye is due to an infectious agent, there may be a yellow or green discharge.

If the condition is caused by an infectious agent, antibiotics are usually prescribed. Because many of the bacteria that cause conjunctivitis can be quite damaging, it is important to see a doctor.

Chamomile Eye Compress

Avoid applying matricaria recutita (German chamomile) essential oil, even well diluted, directly to the eye as the tissue is too sensitive. If you do not have the herb but have the oil, it can be used safely as a wash. Blend 1 drop of German chamomile essential oil and 1 drop of lavender essential oil into a teaspoon (5 mL) of raw honey and apply this blend to the tissue around the eye. Be sure not to apply the blend into the eye itself, although if it is diluted in 1 cup (250 mL) of warm distilled water, it may be used on a cloth as a compress. (Avoid using *raw* honey with children under 1 year of age as it may contain botulinum toxin spores and babies are more susceptible to the effects.)

Matricaria Recutita (German Chamomile) Tea

A tea made from matricaria recutita is an excellent treatment. Brew a cup of tea with two chamomile tea bags and hot, but not boiling, water. Cover the cup and allow the tea to brew until the tea bags come to a tolerable temperature, keeping in mind that the hand perceives heat differently than the tender, inflamed tissue of the eye area. Place one tea bag over the infected eye until it cools, then replace with the other tea bag. Repeat until the tea has cooled completely. If there is a bacterial or viral agent involved, do not apply the tea bag to the other eye, to avoid the spread of infection.

Aromatherapy for Acupoints

Myrtus communis (green myrtle) hydrosol is one of the best aromatherapy treatments for all conditions of the eyes. It is a mild, calming treatment to help soothe the irritation. See the product's packaging for directions on applying it.

Best Acupressure Point for Conjunctivitis
BL1 • Jingming (see Bladder 1, page 49)

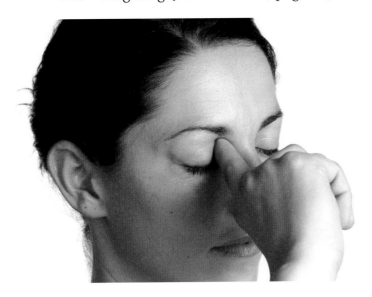

Other Acupressure Points to Consider
After pressing the best acupressure point for this condition, follow with one of these points:

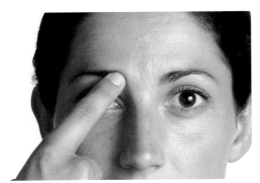

For conjunctivitis with eye pain, add
BL2 • Zanzhu (see Bladder 2, page 50)

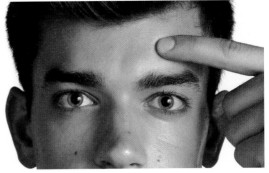

For conjunctivitis with headache, add
GB14 • Yangbai (see Gallbladder 14,
page 68)

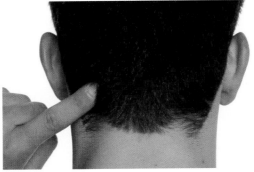

For conjunctivitis with cold symptoms, add
GB20 • Fengchi (see Gallbladder 20,
page 69)

Constipation

While constipation is commonly understood to be slow or difficult bowel movements, medically it is defined as fewer than one complete bowel movement a day. Constipation has many causes. Dehydration and lack of fiber can lead to small, dry stools, a situation more easily addressed by changes in diet. Lack of tone in the bowel, medications, bowel surgery, restricted exercise, dietary sensitivities and age can all result in slower transit time.

Signs and Symptoms

The two most common forms of constipation are a very slow transit time with normal stool or regular movements but with dry, small, pebbly stools. A feeling of incomplete evacuation may accompany a slower transit time. Constipation can lead to a need to strain — a tendency that usually leads to other problems, such as hemorrhoids or rectal bleeding. There is often pain, especially with dry stool.

The act of defecating is moderated by both sympathetic and parasympathetic nerves. If there is an ongoing issue, a patient may experience symptoms related to both nervous systems; for example, sweating and dizziness, and an increase in heart rate.

If the symptoms continue for more than a week, it is probably a good idea to talk with your doctor.

> ## Note
> If there is a complete lack of bowel movement, it may indicate a blockage in the bowel — contact a doctor as soon as possible.

Other Treatments

- Ensure adequate fiber, water and oil in the diet. If the constipation is due to lack of motility rather than dehydration, consider abdominal massage to help the muscles of digestion do their job
- Eat more slippery foods: marshmallow, slippery elm, okra, soaked dried fruit
- Ensure a good intake of probiotics, preferably in the form of cultured vegetables, which also offer fiber and moisture
- Consume digestive bitters or a tablespoon (15 mL) of apple cider vinegar in warm water before meals
- Massage a blend of lavender in St. John's wort oil over the lower abdomen. Castor oil packs may also help
- Avoid dairy for a month to test its sensitivity. Add it back to your diet slowly; if constipation returns, you may have a dairy sensitivity

Aromatherapy for Acupoints

Basil on ST25

With pain: lavender on ST40

With feeling of incompletion: fennel on ST36 with KI3 (bend over and grab both sides of the ankles)

Caution

Be wary of over-the-counter laxatives — using them for extended periods can make the problem worse.

Best Acupressure Point for Constipation

ST25 • Tianshu (see Stomach 25, page 38)

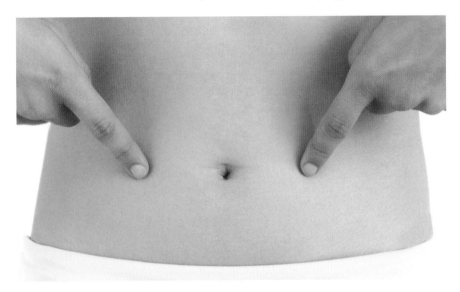

Other Acupressure Points to Consider

After pressing the best acupressure point for this condition, follow with one of these points:

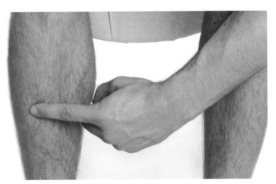

For constipation with pain, add
ST40 • Fenglong (see Stomach 40, page 40)

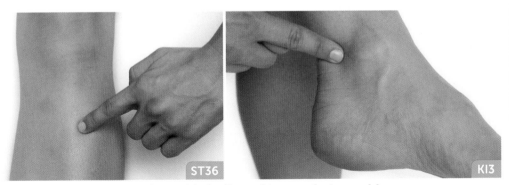

For constipation with feeling of incompletion, add
ST36 • Zusanli (see Stomach 36, page 39) followed by KI3 • Taixi (see Kidney 3, page 55)

Cough

Cough is not actually a condition but a symptom. It is the body's attempt to remove something foreign from the lungs and is characterized by a forceful expulsion of air against the resistance of the diaphragm, which is why prolonged coughing can lead to abdominal pain.

Cough could be a response to an irritant lodged in the airways. It may also occur as the body attempts to expel phlegm-containing infectious agents during a cold or flu. Certain chronic respiratory conditions, such as asthma or bronchitis, are usually associated with cough. Allergies can also bring on cough.

Signs and Symptoms

There are many different types of cough. Those associated with infectious agents usually produce yellow or green phlegm. Allergic cough is characterized by copious, thin to watery clear phlegm. If the cough is extreme, the phlegm may be pink as tiny capillaries in the lungs burst under increased pressure. An unproductive (dry) cough often occurs at the end of a cold or respiratory infection.

Any persistent or debilitating (exhausting) cough, especially in the very young or the elderly, should be examined by a doctor. Extreme cough may lead to torn muscles, prolapsed bladder or other prolapse, and in some cases has actually resulted in broken ribs.

> ## Note
> If there are urinary or bowel changes, or there is a sudden sharp pain in the chest and it does not change, see a doctor.

Other Treatments

- Diffuse into the sick room one drop of each essential oil: rosemary, lemon, eucalyptus and thyme
- Since most coughs are viral, consider adding one drop of Ravintsara into one teaspoon (5 mL) of raw honey, preferably manuka honey. Keep in mind that raw honey should not be used in children under 1 year
- For a cough due to allergies, see page 138
- Marshmallow tea can help encourage secretions in unproductive cough

Aromatherapy for Acupoints

With thin clear to white mucus: pine on CV22

With sticky yellow mucus: eucalyptus globulus on LU7 and peppermint inhaled from a steam bath

With pain in the chest: blue or German chamomile on LR3

Spasmodic cough: marjoram on CV22

Caution

Some cough may be triggered by essential oil treatments, so proceed with caution (see the box on page 105).

Best Acupressure Point for Cough

CV22 • Tiantu (see Conception Vessel 22, page 82)
Also recommended for: spasmodic cough

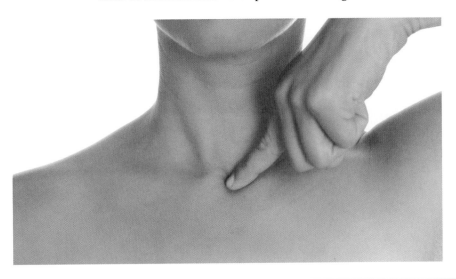

Other Acupressure Points to Consider

After pressing the best acupressure point for this condition, follow with one of these points:

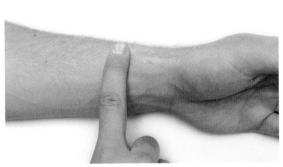

For cough with sticky yellow mucus, add
LU7 • Lieque (see Lung 7, page 25)

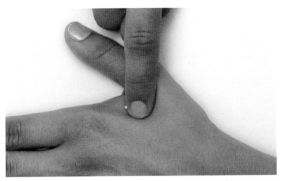

For cough with no mucus, add
LI4 • Hegu (see Large Intestine 4, page 29)

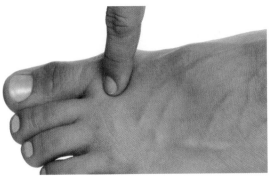

For cough with pain in the chest, add
LR3 • Taichong (see Liver 3, page 74)

Cystitis (Bladder Infections)

Cystitis is an inflammation of the urinary system, specifically the bladder. It is usually the result of an infection, but sometimes there is no obvious cause. In some cases, bladder infections may be caused by nerve damage, an autoimmune reaction or irritants in the diet.

Bladder infections have been attributed to many different bacteria, but the most common is *Escherichia coli (E. coli)*. This infection tends to manifest symptoms in women, likely because of the proximity of the female urethra to the vagina and anus. Sexual intercourse is a common route for transmitting the bacteria into the urinary system. In fact, a nickname for cystitis is "honeymoon infection."

Signs and Symptoms

Cystitis is characterized by increasing pain and urgency as the bladder fills. The pain often radiates to the genitals and anus. There is usually incontinence and the feeling of incomplete evacuation after urination. Itching, cramping and incontinence may all accompany the infection, as well as polyuria (increased frequency of urination). Leukorrhea (vaginal discharge) usually occurs concurrently with the infection.

It is quite common for bladder infections to recur after the first incident. Fortunately, preventive measures may be quite effective at decreasing the likelihood of repeat infections. The treatments outlined here are designed to be preventive and not to treat acute infections, although they may help reduce symptoms.

Other Treatments

- Stopping the stream of urine mid-flow is one of the best exercises to reverse incontinence. Practice this exercise only when not experiencing an active infection
- Yoga has a good track record for helping to strengthen bladder control
- Juniper berry (see box)
- Cranberry juice may prevent the bacteria from adhering to the lining of the urinary tract. D-Mannose works similarly

> ## Aromatherapy for Acupoints
>
> **Bladder infections:** juniper berry or thyme on KI7
>
> **Incontinence:** carrot seed on CV4
>
> **With burning:** blue chamomile or helichrysum on LR3
>
> **Due to prolapse:** orange on GV20

Juniper Berry Tea

Juniper berry is used in medical aromatherapy for kidney infections and will also have benefits for the urinary system. It can be made into a tea with other herbs. Steep in hot water, along with corn silk, dandelion root or parsley.

Best Acupressure Point for Cystitis

KI7 • Fuliu (see Kidney 7, page 57)

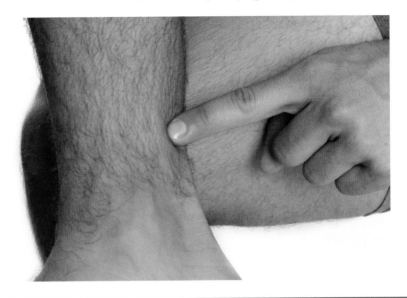

Other Acupressure Points to Consider

After pressing the best acupressure point for this condition, follow with one of these points:

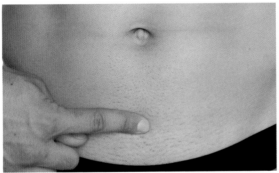

For bladder infections with incontinence, add CV4 • Guanyuan (see Conception Vessel 4, page 78)

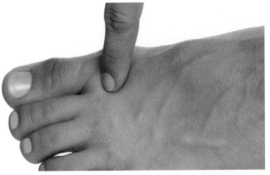

For bladder infections with burning, add LR3 • Taichong (see Liver 3, page 74)

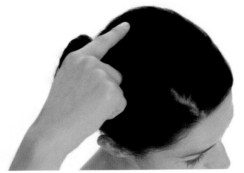

For bladder infections due to prolapse, add GV20 • Baihui (see Governing Vessel 20, page 84)

Depression

Depression is considered a mental emotional disorder wherein the symptoms overwhelm the capacity to live a typical life — which varies from patient to patient.

The incidence of depression is on the rise, as many find it difficult to navigate a rapidly changing world. There is often a triggering event, such as an unexpected change of circumstances (divorce, death, a troubling medical diagnosis), or it may develop idiopathically (no known cause). Some bouts of depression are short-lived and may happen in isolation, but this is the exception. Many people suffer from depression for life; however, recent treatment plans have helped patients manage the disease so it is no longer so debilitating.

Vitamin deficiencies are commonly seen with depression, and supplementing may resolve this issue. One type of depression, seasonal affective disorder (SAD), is triggered by a lack of sunlight. Diet plays a huge role in depression — one study links increased sugar consumption with increased depression and a greater consumption of fruit and vegetables with decreased symptoms.

Some medications, including many that treat depression, caution that depression may be a side effect. Corticosteroids, barbiturates and opiates have long been associated with depression and often lead to a rebound effect of worsened depression.

Signs and Symptoms

Most commonly, those with depression experience exhaustion, lack of energy for daily activities and no inclination to engage with society and life in general. There are often physical symptoms as well, such as decreased or increased appetite, digestive changes and body weakness or heaviness, among others. Decreased oxygen to the brain can be a depressant, so respiratory conditions may be accompanied by depression.

Aromatherapy for Acupoints

Lemon balm on Ht7

Lack of faith: frankincense on KI9

Due to exhaustion: black spruce on ST40

Due to anger: rose, chamomile or helichrysum on LR2

Note

Depression can manifest as mild to extreme. People who experience extreme symptoms may be considered at risk of committing suicide. If a person is experiencing extreme symptoms, it is very important that they seek professional help. The suggestions here may help manage milder symptoms.

Other Treatments

- Beneficial supplements include B vitamins, vitamin D, SAM-e (S-adenosylmethionine), magnesium, 5-HTP, fish oil and holy basil

Best Acupressure Point for Depression

Ht7 • Shenmen (see Heart 7, page 46)

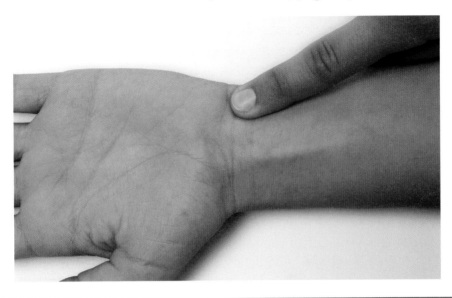

Other Acupressure Points to Consider

After pressing the best acupressure point for this condition, follow with one of these points:

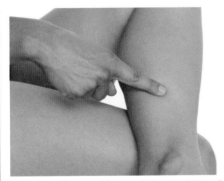

For depression with a crisis of faith or spirit, add KI9 • Zhubin (see Kidney 9, page 58)

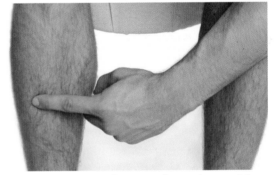

For depression due to exhaustion, add ST40 • Fenglong (see Stomach 40, page 40)

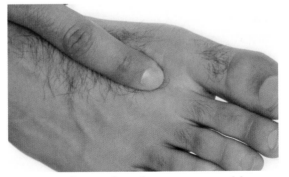

For depression due to anger, add LR2 • Xingjian (see Liver 2, page 73)

Diabetes

Diabetes is a blood sugar dysregulation due to changes in the pancreas. In particular, the body is not able to produce enough insulin, the substance that processes sugar. If there is not enough insulin, the sugar does not make its way into the cells but instead remains in the bloodstream, leading to high sugar levels.

Type 1 diabetes usually develops in childhood and is an autoimmune disease in which the immune system attacks the beta cells of the pancreas, the cells responsible for producing insulin, destroying them in the process. Patients with type 1 diabetes are completely dependent on insulin injections.

Type 2 diabetes is defined by insulin resistance, leading to initial increases in insulin, but eventually it can lead to pancreatic failure and the need for insulin injections. Poor dietary choices and obesity are often causes. Type 2 is often preceded by metabolic syndrome, which is a risk factor for both diabetes and heart disease.

Gestational diabetes may arise during pregnancy. This is a serious complication so all mothers are tested during pregnancy.

Signs and Symptoms

The most common symptoms in both type 1 and later-stage type 2 are obvious yet contrary. For example, there is increased hunger but weight loss is common as the cells are starved of the sugar they need to function. Increased thirst will lead to increased fluid intake, but dehydration can occur.

Tingling is common due to changes in nerve cells. As the blood vessels also change, the blood becomes less able to deliver oxygen to the cells. The extremities may develop frequent infections as the blood becomes less efficient at delivering white blood cells around the body. There may be changes in vision.

> ## Note
> Diabetic shock is an extreme and dangerous situation, characterized by dizziness, mental confusion, tremors and rapid breathing. There is a characteristically fruity scent on the breath. This is an emergency situation and should be treated immediately. The suggestions here are to help manage the milder symptoms of diabetes.

Other Treatments
- Magnesium and chromium picolinate; CoQ10
- Cinnamon capsules
- Seeds such as fenugreek, coriander and dill to improve insulin receptivity. Add these to the diet or consider capsules

Aromatherapy for Acupoints

Eucalyptus citriodora on SP6

Numbness and tingling at the extremities: geranium on LU7

With edema: juniper berry on SP10

With cold feet: rosemary on SP4

Best Acupressure Point for Diabetes

SP6 • Sanyinjiao (see Spleen 6, page 43)

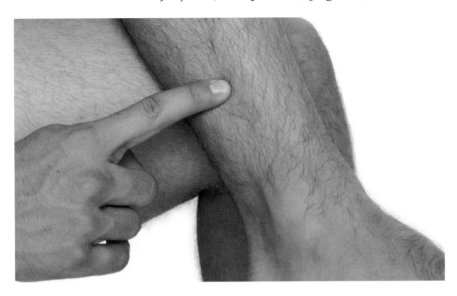

Other Acupressure Points to Consider

After pressing the best acupressure point for this condition, follow with one of these points:

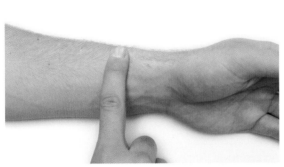

For diabetes with numbness and tingling at the extremities, add LU7 • Lieque (see Lung 7, page 25)

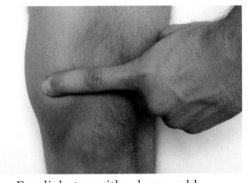

For diabetes with edema, add SP10 • Xuehai (see Spleen 10, page 45)

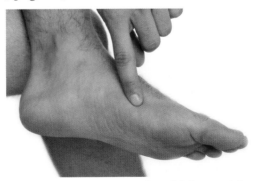

For diabetes with cold feet, add SP4 • Gongsun (see Spleen 4, page 42)

Diarrhea

While diarrhea is commonly understood as stool that is loose to watery, medically speaking, diarrhea is defined as an increase in bowel movements that have less consistency, or regular frequency but looser consistency. Diarrhea is a symptom of many acute and chronic diseases. Bacterial and viral infections are the most common cause of acute diarrhea, but stress, food sensitivities and malabsorption, Crohn's disease, irritable bowel syndrome (IBS) and ulcerative colitis are all culprits. Gastrointestinal (GI) infections, like those caused by *Clostridium difficile*, may lead to life-threatening diarrhea where patients experience more than 10 watery stools a day. This can lead to severe electrolyte imbalance, among other symptoms.

Diarrhea is the body's natural response to poisoning, from alcohol or over-medicating, for example, as an attempt to purge the irritant.

Signs and Symptoms

The main sign is an increased number of bowel movements; specifically, more than three a day. Bowel movements may be loose to watery or foamy. Diarrhea is often accompanied by cramping or other GI pain. There may also be a sensation of heat, dizziness, nausea or sweating. Short-term weakness often occurs with acute diarrhea, whereas a chronic case can be debilitating.

Notes

If the stool contains mucus or blood, it may a sign of a more serious condition. Stay hydrated while diarrhea continues! Contact a physician if diarrhea is ongoing for more than 48 hours (sooner in small children, the elderly or convalescing patients) because dehydration is a very serious consequence and intravenous fluids may be necessary.

Other Treatments

• Suppositories, enemas (see box)
• Cinnamon and oregano capsules for infectious diarrhea
• Essential oils rich in phenols have a history of benefit in the gut — oregano, spearmint, thyme, basil, bay, cinnamon and clove. Add these oils to foods or eat fresh as herbs

Treating with Astringing Enemas

Enemas are an excellent route of delivery for chronic diarrhea. They help to tone the tissue, which helps with slowing the transit time, as well as possibly killing the pathogen causing the diarrhea. Diluted apple cider vinegar is one option.

Aromatherapy for Acupoints

Orange on CV12

With cramping: fennel on CV12

With cold sensation: cinnamon on SP8

With hot sensation: rose or lavender on LI11

With colitis: rosemary verbenone on ST25

Best Acupressure Point for Diarrhea

CV12 • Zhongwan (see Conception Vessel 12, page 80)

Also recommended for: diarrhea with cramping

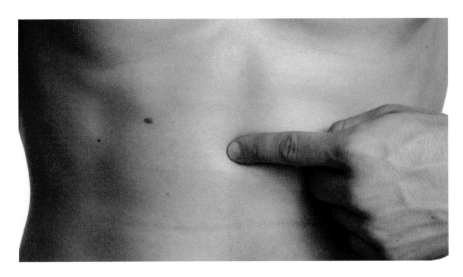

Other Acupressure Points to Consider

After pressing the best acupressure point for this condition, follow with one of these points:

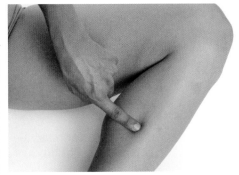

For diarrhea with cold sensation, add
SP8 • Diji (see Spleen 8, page 44)

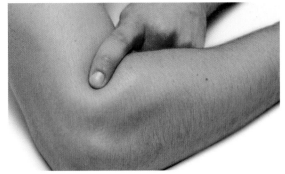

For diarrhea with hot sensation, add
LI11 • Quchi (see Large Intestine 11, page 31)

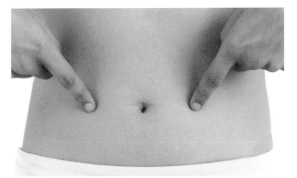

For diarrhea with colitis, add
ST25 • Tianshu (see Stomach 25, page 38)

Edema

Edema occurs when fluid from the circulatory system leaks out and pools in the interstices (spaces between structures in the body). This can be a natural and appropriate response to an injury or infection — swollen tissue is a sign that the immune system is delivering white blood cells to help repair the problem. In this case, edema naturally reduces as the repair is completed. Allergic reactions are another example of this kind of edema.

Edema may also be a symptom of systems failing due to age or illness, as in the case of congestive heart failure, liver failure or renal failure. Many medications list edema as a possible side effect, including corticosteroids and NSAIDs. Obesity can bring on edema because many of the body's systems are under undue strain from the excess weight. Lymphedema, due to faulty lymphatic drainage, is usually associated with cancer and the removal of lymph nodes.

Signs and Symptoms

Swollen, soft, boggy tissues are signs of edema. Edema associated with inflammation is usually accompanied with heat and redness, and fades relatively quickly. Edematous tissue resulting from more serious illnesses may appear pale and feel cooler and clammy — with pitting edema, tissue that is pressed maintains an indentation after removing the pressure.

> ## Note
> Unilateral edema occurring in one lower leg may indicate a DVT (deep vein thrombosis), a potentially life-threatening condition. Edema in the mouth and throat tissue following a food allergy is also a more serious and potentially life-threatening response, as the swelling can block airways. Pulmonary edema is another serious condition that can lead to reduced oxygen levels.

Other Treatments

- Grapefruit topical dilution over areas of edema — apply gently
- Gentle exercise. The body moves blood and lymph back to the heart and lungs for reoxygenation through the action of muscles on the veins and lymph nodes
- Massage — light strokes performed by a specialist in lymphatic drainage
- Foods that reduce edema include beets, garlic, grapes, leafy greens, leeks, onions, parsley and pumpkin. Many of these are high in potassium, a mineral depleted by diuretics
- Alpha-lipoic acid (ALA), vitamin C

Aromatherapy for Acupoints

With cold: fennel on SP6

In the upper body: cypress on ST43

In the lower body: juniper on KI7

Caution

When applying dilutions or massage over areas of edema, do not apply with vigorous strokes. Edema results when the body is unable to process the fluids fast enough to keep them in the bloodstream. Overly vigorous application places greater stress on the already overburdened circulatory and urinary systems.

Best Acupressure Point for Edema
SP6 • Sanyinjiao (see Spleen 6, page 43)

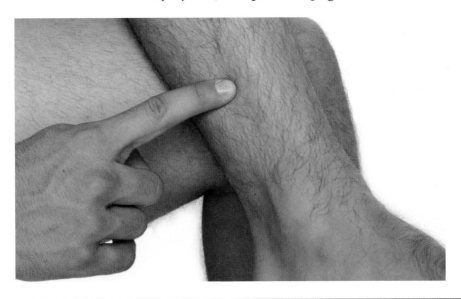

Other Acupressure Points to Consider

After pressing the best acupressure point for this condition, follow with one of these points:

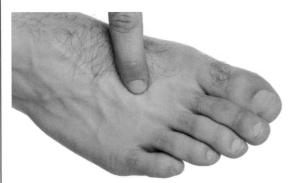

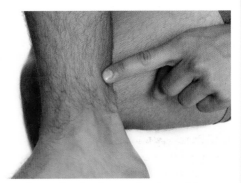

For edema in the upper body, add
ST43 • Xiangu (see Stomach 43, page 41)

For edema in the lower body, add
KI7 • Fuliu (see Kidney 7, page 57)

Epicondylitis (Tennis Elbow, Golfer's Elbow)

Epicondylitis is the name given to pain that occurs in the elbow. It usually occurs from overuse, or repetitive actions; swinging a racquet or club is a common cause, as the name suggests. In truth, it is often seen in those not playing either sport — mechanics, factory workers, professional cleaners and weavers regularly develop epicondylitis.

With this condition, repetition further irritates already inflamed tissues. The condition may be due to inflammation in the muscles or tendons, or both. Tennis elbow happens when the lateral (outer) side is painful, and golfer's elbow occurs on the medial (inner) side.

Signs and Symptoms

Pain is the primary — and in many cases only — symptom. The pain is usually a constant ache, exacerbated by the same motions that led to the condition. The pain is worse with gripping, lifting or twisting; for example, opening a jar may be painful. Stiffness and a significant decrease in range of motion are common. If the tendon or muscle is torn, the joint may be entirely out of commission.

Continued use with no rest will aggravate the problem. It is crucial to stop the activity that led to the problem so tissues can heal, although this can be difficult if the activities are part of daily living or one's work.

Other Treatments

- Adequate rest, particularly for the part of the body concerned
- Glucosamine chondroitin, hyaluronic acid, anti-inflammatory blends with ginger and turmeric
- Vitamins A and C

Aromatherapy for Acupoints

Tennis elbow: pain blend (see page 136) and carrot seed on LI11

Golfer's elbow: add a drop of the blend above to the opposite side of the elbow and hold both sides at one time.

Radiating down the arm: helichrysum on TW3

Radiating up the arm: pain blend (see page 136) and carrot seed on TW14

Best Acupressure Point for Epicondylitis

LI11 • Quchi (see Large Intestine 11, page 31)

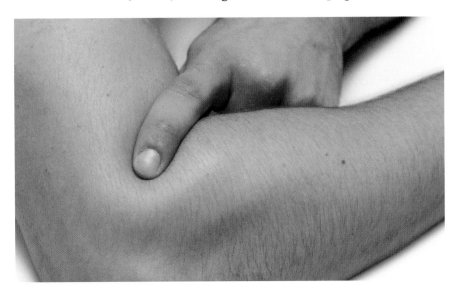

Other Acupressure Points to Consider

After pressing the best acupressure point for this condition, follow with one of these points:

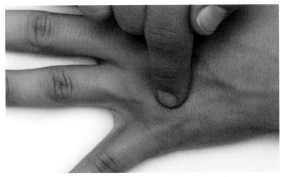

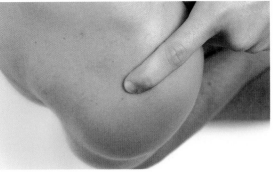

For epicondylitis radiating down the arm, add TW3 • Zhongzhu (see Triple Warmer 3, page 63)

For epicondylitis radiating up the arm, add TW14 • Jianliao (see Triple Warmer 14, page 64)

Fungal Infections

Fungal infections can happen nearly anywhere in or on the body. The most common infections occur topically — on the skin or nails, for example. Fungal eye infections are also fairly common.

As is the case with most infectious agents, the same fungi that can lead to infection exist harmlessly all around us but can cause issues when the body is compromised. Fungal infections are more common in people with compromised immune function because of disease or immunosuppressant drugs.

Fungal infections occur when the body is infected by spores of many different kinds of fungi. Some spores occur more regionally; for example, the coccidioides fungus is known to occur in the southwestern United States.

Candida is the causative agent in yeast infections. These most commonly occur vaginally but can happen anywhere; thrush, for example, is a candida fungal infection of the throat.

Signs and Symptoms

Itching, burning rash, often with raised lesions, is a common symptom. The skin becomes more irritated and sensitive as the infection progresses, leading to flaking, cracked skin. If the fungal infection occurs on mucous membranes, there is usually discharge.

Fungal infections are notoriously hard to resolve. It takes diligent application of antifungals to see results, and even natural antifungal agents are hard on healthy tissue. If the skin is already irritated and cracked, the treatments may worsen the situation. The suggestions here are to help reduce symptoms of the infection and eradicate the fungus, but if the irritation worsens, consider a different approach.

> ### Note
> Respiratory fungal infections, such as pneumocystis pneumonia, usually occur in immune-compromised people and can be quite dangerous. Seek medical attention.

Other Treatments

- Clove dilution gargle for thrush
- Tea tree suppositories are effective against more stubborn infections
- Eucalyptus and peppermint oils have all been shown to be effective against many different fungi

Aromatherapy for Acupoints

Thrush: rose geranium on CV23

Tinea: geranium, lemongrass and patchouli on LU9

Nail fungus: cinnamon, thyme and niaouli on LU11

Vaginal candida (mild infections): geranium on CV1

Tinea

Tinea is another fungus that regularly causes infection. The most common are Tinea pedis (athlete's foot), Tinea cruris (jock itch), Tinea capitis (ringworm on the head) and Tinea corporis (ringworm of the body). If the infection is caused by tinea, it may take on a ring shape, although this is not always the case.

Best Acupressure Point for Fungal Infections

SP6 • Sanyinjiao (see Spleen 6, page 43)

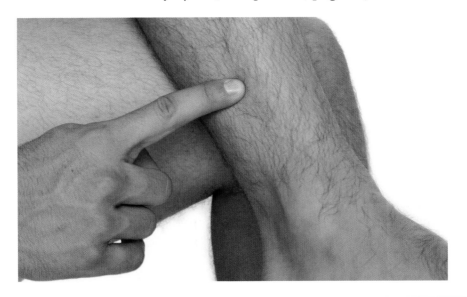

Other Acupressure Points to Consider

After pressing the best acupressure point for this condition, follow with one of these points:

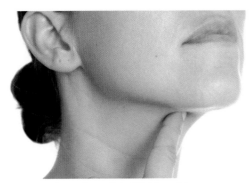

For thrush, add CV23 • Lianquan (see Conception Vessel 23, page 83)

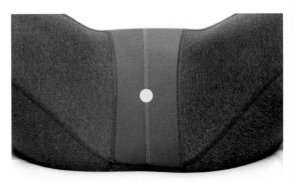

For vaginal candida, add CV1 • Huiyin (see Conception Vessel 1, page 76)

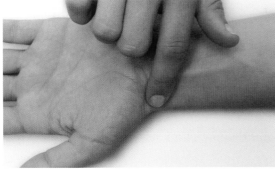

For tinea, add LU9 • Taiyuan (see Lung 9, page 26)

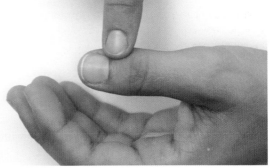

For nail fungus, add LU11 • Shaoshang (see Lung 11, page 28)

GERD (Heartburn, Acid Reflux)

Often referred to as GERD (gastroesophageal reflux disease) or by its common names, heartburn, or acid reflux, is the condition of stomach acid flowing back through the lower esophageal sphincter and into the esophagus and throat, causing burning and irritation.

Most commonly associated with stress, acid reflux can be triggered by foods, medications, anxiety or other triggers. Often the condition will aggravate itself — as the acid rises, the tender tissue of the esophagus will create a thickened area for protection. While it prevents damage to the tissue, this thickening will also cause the lower esophageal sphincter to become even less effective. Individuals with hiatal hernia often experience GERD as a symptom — as the stomach pushes up through the lower esophageal sphincter, it is no longer able to close off the stomach from the esophagus, which results in increased stomach acid outside of the stomach.

Signs and Symptoms

Most commonly, the symptoms are a burning or foul taste in the mouth. There may also be burning and pain in the esophagus, which is often felt in the chest. Usually these symptoms arise fairly quickly after encountering a trigger. There is diminished desire for food or drink because they will exacerbate the symptoms. Some people experience an increase in salivation when reflux is triggered.

> ### Note
> The symptoms listed above often mimic the symptoms of a myocardial infarction (heart attack). Be sure to see a doctor if the symptoms do not change or get worse.

Other Treatments

- Orange peel capsules. Take as needed, up to several times a day (check directions on package)
- Peppermint capsules. Some people get relief from them, while others find they worsen symptoms. Try a cup of peppermint tea first or try the fennel and orange peel tea (see box)

Aromatherapy for Acupoints

Grapefruit on CV12

With spasm: tarragon on CV22

With nausea: peppermint on PC6

With bloating: fennel on ST36

With chest pain: blue chamomile on CV17

Fennel and Orange Peel Tea

This tea can help alleviate symptoms of GERD. To make your own, add a few strips of orange peel and 1 teaspoon (5 mL) fennel seeds to a cup of hot water. Let steep for a few minutes, until peel and seeds settle to the bottom, and sip.

Best Acupressure Point for GERD

CV12 • Zhongwan (see Conception Vessel 12, page 80)

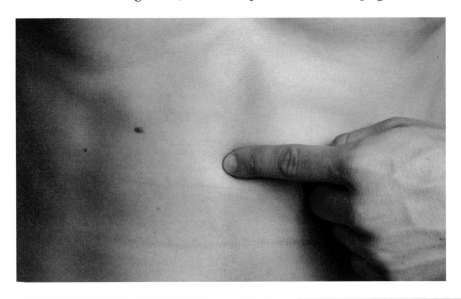

Other Acupressure Points to Consider

After pressing the best acupressure point for this condition, follow with one of these points:

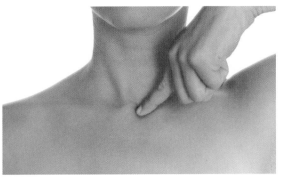

For heartburn with spasm, add
CV22 • Tiantu (see Conception Vessel 22, page 82)

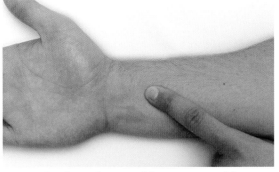

For heartburn with nausea, add
PC6 • Neiguan (see Pericardium 6, page 61)

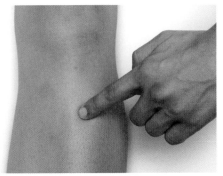

For heartburn with bloating, add
ST36 • Zusanli (see Stomach 36, page 39)

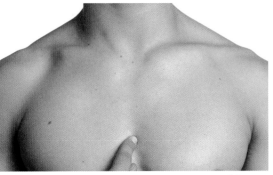

For heartburn with chest pain, add
CV17 • Tanzhong (see Conception Vessel 17, page 81)

Halitosis (Bad Breath)

The most common causes are infection and poor digestion. The infection may be associated with poor oral hygiene or gum disease; specifically, pockets of infection that form between the teeth and gums may harbor bacteria. This leads to inflammation and tissue degradation. The gums are particularly susceptible to infection.

Infection could also be happening lower in the gastrointestinal tract. Ulcers and acid reflux create a distinctive odor. Sjogren's syndrome or other conditions that lead to dry mouth, and lung conditions like bronchitis, postnasal drip or pneumonia, all result in odor. Thrush, an oral yeast infection, can lead to bad breath as well. Many prescription drugs may lead to halitosis. Smoking and dehydration worsen the situation.

Signs and Symptoms

Foul odor from the mouth is of course the most common symptom. There may be dry mouth, or pain if the source is inflammation and infection. The condition can lead to social isolation if it is severe enough.

Aromatherapy for Acupoints

Tooth decay: black pepper on LI5

Thrush: rose geranium on CV23

Sinus infection: eucalyptus globulus on LI20

GI imbalance: fennel on CV12

Note

Bad breath can be a symptom of a serious condition, so finding the root cause is important. Halitosis may be a result of narrowed blood vessels to the gums and may be a sign of an underlying circulatory condition, heart disease or diabetes.

Other Treatments

- Flossing or using an interdental brush to clear food particles that lead to inflammation and stimulate blood flow to the gums
- Using a mouthwash (see Toothache, page 246)
- Oil pulling (see page 146)
- Treating gut imbalance with probiotics, cultured foods, enzymes

Best Acupressure Point for Halitosis

CV23 • Lianquan (see Conception Vessel 23, page 83)

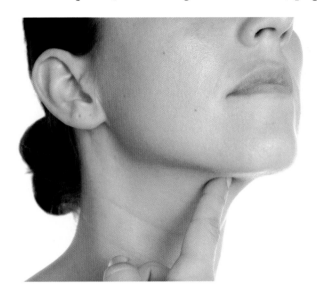

Other Acupressure Points to Consider

After pressing the best acupressure point for this condition, follow with one of these points:

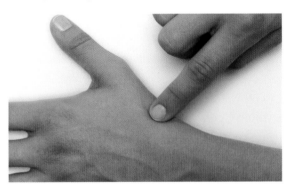

For halitosis with tooth decay, add
LI5 • Yangxi (see Large Intestine 5,
page 30)

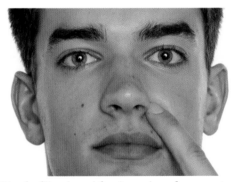

For halitosis with sinus involvement, add
LI20 • Yingxiang (see Large Intestine 20,
page 33)

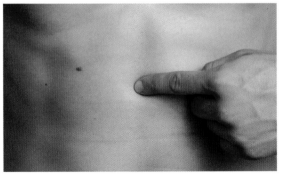

For halitosis with poor digestion, add
CV12 • Zhongwan (see Conception
Vessel 12, page 80)

Headache

The different types of headache define areas where the pain is experienced (such as frontal or occipital) or point to the different causes (tension, for example).

Frontal headaches are felt mostly in the forehead. Temporal headaches can occur anywhere along the side of the head. Occipital headaches are felt along the occiput, the bony ridge at the back of the head. Tension headaches usually occur in a band around the head, and vertex headaches are felt at the top of the head. Cluster headaches appear in the same spot again and again, but usually each episode does not last long. They are one-sided and often occur around or behind the eye.

Sinus infection and toothache can also cause headaches, as can eye strain. Most headaches are due in part to changes in blood flow to the head. These can be due to structural changes; for example, headaches that result from injury and swelling. Dehydration may also be a cause. Lack of sleep, diet and dietary change — such as reducing sugar or caffeine — stress and medications have all been implicated in the onset of headache.

Signs and Symptoms

Pain is of course the main symptom, but other symptoms may vary and include irritability, inability to focus, dizziness (especially with migraine headaches), nausea and vomiting. Some headaches are associated with a different set of symptoms with each presentation; specifically, migraine sufferers may experience extreme light sensitivity, visual changes and little pain, or the pain may be so severe that they retreat from life for a few days. Typically, the neck and shoulders are involved.

Note
Headaches can be a sign of a more serious condition. If they occur with increasing frequency or intensity, visit your doctor. If vision changes occur, it may be an emergency situation. Migraine headaches are unique and should be diagnosed by a doctor. The sudden onset of an excruciating headache is probably an emergency situation.

Other Treatments
• A mustard footbath, along with a peppermint compress on the back of the neck, can work wonders

Aromatherapy for Acupoints

Lavender-peppermint blend (see box) on LI4 and on any recommended acupressure point.

Wintergreen or birch on any recommended acupressure point.

Caution
Wintergreen or birch essential oil may cause an allergic reaction in those with salicylate allergies.

Headache Blend

Add 3 tablespoons (15 mL) of jojoba oil to an empty small bottle. Add 1 drop of peppermint essential oil. Slowly add lavender essential oil, 1 drop at a time. Sniff after each drop until you can detect both scents (around 8 to 12 drops of lavender). The final blend varies for each person.

Best Acupressure Point for Headache

LI4 • Hegu (see Large Intestine 4, page 29)

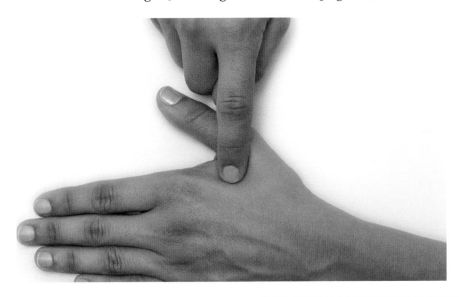

Other Acupressure Points to Consider

After pressing the best acupressure point for this condition, follow with one of these points:

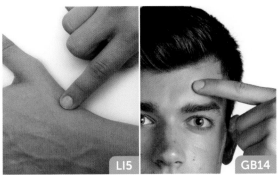

For frontal headache, add LI5 • Yangxi
(see Large Intestine 5, page 30) or GB14 •
Yangbai (see Gallbladder 14, page 68)

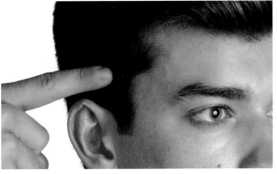

For one-sided headache, add
GB6 • Xuanli (see Gallbladder 6, page 67)

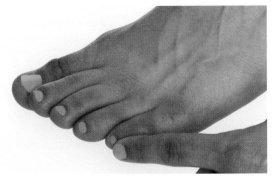

For apex headache, add
BL67 • Zhiyin (see Bladder 67, page 53)

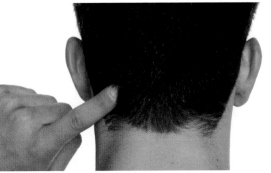

For temporal headache, add
GB20 • Fengchi (see Gallbladder 20,
page 69)

Hepatitis

Hepatitis is liver inflammation, usually caused by the hepatitis virus. It can be caused by alcoholism and an autoimmune imbalance. Hepatitis means inflammation (-itis) of the liver (hepa). Inflammation of the liver can be caused by a virus (confusingly named after the symptom it causes). Hepatitis may also result from alcoholism or an autoimmune attack. If it is caused by the virus, the disease may be spread to others through contact with the blood of an infected person.

Hepatitis viruses come in many types, but the three most common are Hep A, Hep B and Hep C.

Hepatitis A (Hep A or HAV) is transmitted by the fecal-oral route. It is acute and a short-lived relative to the other types.

Hepatitis B (Hep B or HBV) is transmitted by blood or other bodily fluids. It can lead to chronic liver disease if not treated.

Hepatitis C (Hep C or HCV) is also spread by blood or other body fluids and manifests many of the same symptoms. It is often associated with intravenous drug use, although some cases are passed on from blood transfusions. It can be passed from mother to child during childbirth and breastfeeding, although this risk is small.

Signs and Symptoms

Hep A mostly results in gastrointestinal distress, such as loss of appetite, nausea, bloating and fatigue. Hep B has an average incubation period of 120 days and may manifest with no symptoms or with jaundice, darkened urine, nausea and vomiting, pain and fatigue. If it develops into a chronic condition, the symptoms linger and get worse. Hep C has a shorter incubation period, about 45 days, and usually appears similarly to Hep B, with mostly the same symptoms. If it develops into a chronic situation, the symptoms worsen and often lead to cirrhosis or liver cancer.

> ## Note
> If there is unexpected weight loss and unexplained digestive changes, seek a medical diagnosis.

Other Treatments

- Dandelion root, licorice and milk thistle as a tea is both reparative and antiviral
- Artichoke promotes bile and helps the liver flush
- Avoid alcohol, which further damages the liver

Aromatherapy for Acupoints

Carrot seed on LR3

With pain:
helichrysum on LR2

Acute Hep A:
fennel on CV12

Best Acupressure Point for Hepatitis

LR3 • Taichong (see Liver 3, page 74)

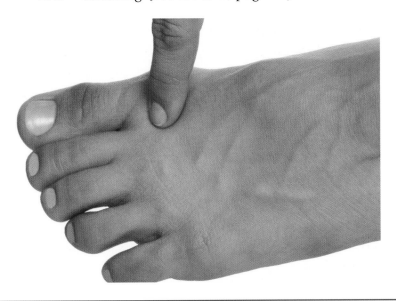

Other Acupressure Points to Consider

After pressing the best acupressure point for this condition, follow with one of these points:

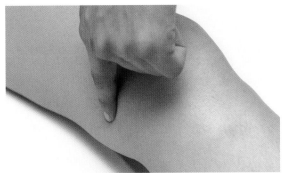

For acute onset symptoms (nausea, vomiting, diarrhea), add LR8 • Ququan (see Liver 8, page 75)

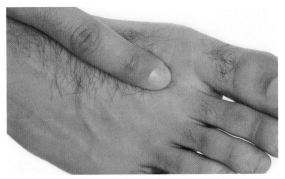

For hepatitis with pain, add LR2 • Xingjian (see Liver 2, page 73)

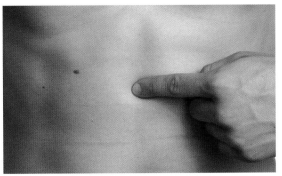

For acute Hep A, add CV12 • Zhongwan (see Conception Vessel 12, page 80)

Hiccup

Hiccup is spasm of the diaphragm that causes a characteristic sound. Eating too much or not eating enough can both lead to hiccups, as can excessive alcohol intake. Smoking may exacerbate a bout of the hiccups. In some people, the condition may arise in stressful situations. The vagus nerve innervates the diaphragm and thus lies at the root of the problem — diseases of the central nervous system may have hiccup as a symptom.

Signs and Symptoms

The condition itself is the main symptom. While the condition is mostly harmless, extended bouts of hiccupping can lead to pain, acid reflux, nausea, vomiting, diaphragmatic cramp and exhaustion. In extreme situations, long-term cases (called intractable hiccup) or intense hiccuping may be fatal.

Diffuse esophageal spasm, or DES, can feel like very painful hiccups, but it is a serious condition associated with many different triggers. Eating the first bite of a meal very slowly may help stop the spasm from happening. Peppermint oil capsules may help, but see a doctor if the symptoms do not abate.

Other Treatments

- Fresh peppermint and tarragon leaves can be added to meals or chewed before meals to reduce the likelihood of hiccup
- Lemon juice and sugar both have a history of folk use to stop hiccup

Hiccup Remedy

One drop of peppermint or tarragon essential oils may be added to 1 teaspoon (5 mL) of honey or olive oil and held in the mouth for a few seconds before swallowing, especially before meals, to prevent or reduce hiccup. Be sure to mix well first.

Aromatherapy for Acupoints

Tarragon on LU10

With pain: Roman chamomile on CV12

Before meals: tarragon on CV23

From alcohol: carrot seed on LR2

Best Acupressure Point for Hiccup

LU10 • Yuji (see Lung 10, page 27)

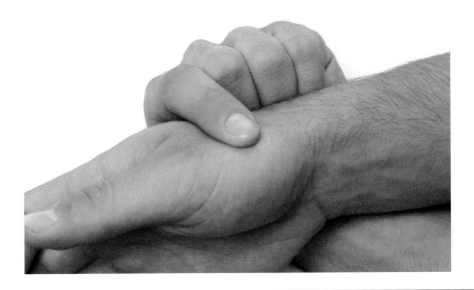

Other Acupressure Points to Consider

After pressing the best acupressure point for this condition, follow with one of these points:

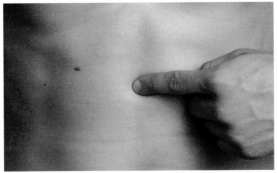

For hiccup with pain, add
CV12 • Zhongwan (see Conception
Vessel 12, page 80)

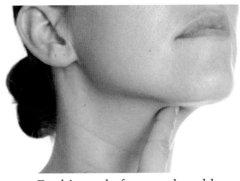

For hiccup before meals, add
CV23 • Lianquan (see Conception
Vessel 23, page 83)

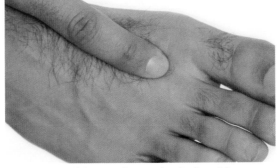

For hiccup from alcohol, add
LR2 • Xingjian (see Liver 2, page 73)

Indigestion

Indigestion mostly describes the pain or discomfort that occurs when there is difficulty digesting foods. It has nearly as many causes as there are cases; for example, it may occur as a reaction to certain foods, because of a lack of specific digestive enzymes, during a microbial infection, because of bad food or poor food combinations, from injury, surgery, stress and more. In addition, other digestive diseases often exhibit indigestion as a symptom.

Signs and Symptoms

Cramping, stabbing, shooting or dull pain in the abdomen, gas and bloating, diarrhea, nausea, vomiting and acid reflux are common symptoms. Some may also experience irritability or fatigue.

While indigestion seems relatively benign, in some cases it may be a sign of a more serious condition. Alcoholism can lead to indigestion, as can drug abuse, mental health conditions, ulcers, gastric diseases and tumors.

Other Treatments

- Cultured foods with digestive enzymes and probiotics from fermented vegetables, kefir or other sources. If these are not available, probiotic capsules or powder from whole food sources may help
- Avoid foods that lead to indigestion — elimination diets can help determine culprit foods
- Abdominal massage (see box)

Aromatherapy for Acupoints

Grapefruit on SP4

With abdominal pain: fennel on CV10

With acid reflux: orange on CV22

With food stagnation in the gut: basil on CV12

Abdominal Massage

Lie on your left side. Starting at the lower right quadrant (near the top of the right hip bone), slowly and gently massage around the abdomen, in small circular motions, moving up the right side, across under the ribs and down the left side until the discomfort is relieved. Using a drop of peppermint essential oil dilution really helps.

Best Acupressure Point for Indigestion
SP4 • Gongsun (see Spleen 4, page 42)

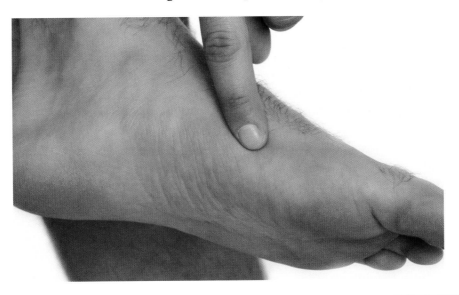

Other Acupressure Points to Consider

After pressing the best acupressure point for this condition, follow with one of these points:

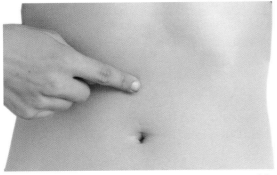

For indigestion with abdominal pain, add CV10 • Xiawan (see Conception Vessel 10, page 79)

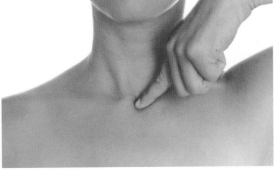

For indigestion with acid reflux, add CV22 • Tiantu (see Conception Vessel 22, page 82)

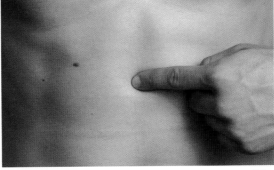

For indigestion with food stagnation, add CV12 • Zhongwan (see Conception Vessel 12, page 80)

Infertility

Infertility is an inability to conceive, specifically after 1 year of unprotected sex. There is no specific or known cause for this condition.

Signs and Symptoms

Symptoms vary in both presentation and severity from couple to couple, but the primary sign is of course lack of pregnancy. For the woman, there may be associated menstrual problems — especially irregular periods that lead to irregular or absent ovulation — due to hormonal imbalances. Other signs that point to a hormonal imbalance include dry skin, weight gain or unexplained mood changes. There may be a blockage in the Fallopian tube. In the male partner, infertility may be the result of erectile difficulties or premature ejaculation. Infertility in males is commonly traced to a low sperm count. Low blood sugar or fatigue may play a role, too. The possibility of a reproductive system tumor also exists in both partners.

Many couples experience deep distress, which predictably leads to greater difficulty in conceiving. Conventional medicine offers artificial insemination and in vitro fertilization, which are often effective at overcoming some of the blocks to becoming pregnant. Natural medicine systems offer great hope, because diet and lifestyle changes can make a big difference. Acupuncture specifically has a history of helping with infertility.

Another important consideration is when to stop trying to become pregnant and consider other options. Pouring energy and hope into repeated attempts that are unsuccessful can significantly and negatively affect health and a relationship.

One of the best home treatments for infertility is to encourage a sense of relaxation and calm while trying to conceive. Using acupoints and essential oils can be very helpful in this regard.

Other Treatments

Women:
- A tea of nettles, red raspberry leaves and red clover is a classic formula to improve fertility and balance hormones
- Essential fatty acids are very important, as are vitamins D and C
- Folate and B vitamins are also valuable

Men:
- Avoid tight underpants and trousers. Avoid hot tubs or hot baths. Heat can damage sperm
- Vitamin C and zinc are helpful for sperm motility
- Supplement with the amino acid arginine, essential fatty acids and vitamins E and B_{12}

Aromatherapy for Acupoints

Clary sage on LR8

Lavender on SP6

Helichrysum on SP10

Women: rose geranium on CV4

Men: rosemary on KI6

Best Acupressure Point for Infertility

CV4 • Guanyuan (see Conception Vessel 4, page 78)

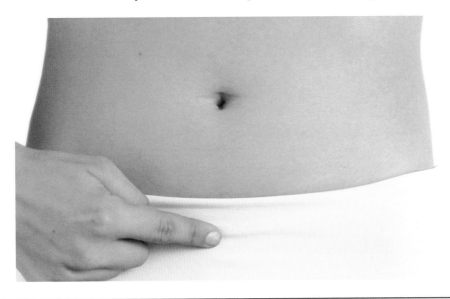

Other Acupressure Points to Consider

After pressing the best acupressure point for this condition, follow with one of these points:

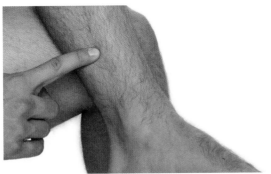

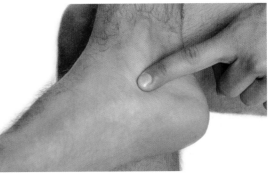

For infertility with sensations of cold, add SP6 • Sanyinjiao (see Spleen 6, page 43)

For infertility due to low sperm count, add KI6 • Zhaohai (see Kidney 6, page 56)

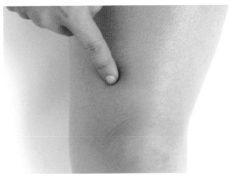

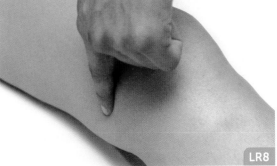

For infertility with bleeding problems, add SP10 • Xuehai (see Spleen 10, page 45) followed by LR8 • Ququan (see Liver 8, page 75)

Insomnia

Insomnia is a disrupted sleep cycle and can present as trouble falling asleep or trouble staying asleep. There are many different reasons why this condition arises, such as stress, anxiety, diet, stimulation, hormonal imbalances, dreams and more.

Signs and Symptoms

Symptoms vary in both presentation and severity from person to person. There may be fatigue or there may be restlessness. Some insomniacs have long stretches of sleeplessness, while others may sleep in short, insufficient blocks of time with short periods of waking in between.

The body's levels of cortisol and melatonin throughout the day form a cycle that determines how we sleep. If either level is out of balance, insomnia will result — and these cycles can be influenced by our behavior choices.

Lack of sleep usually results in irritability and decreased attention or focus. Driving may be impaired if insomnia is extreme. If the condition is chronic, health may generally deteriorate as the body is denied long, uninterrupted sleep, the period of the sleep cycle when the body usually takes care of repair and maintenance.

Other Treatments

- Passionflower capsules for restless exhaustion
- Scullcap capsules for inability to stop thinking
- Hops capsules if worry is causing the insomnia
- California poppy capsules for body tension
- Melatonin supplements to reset the clock
- Valerian, a commonly recommended herb for insomnia, is not useful for about 25% of the population

Aromatherapy for Acupoints

Insomnia: orange and spikenard on GB20 (or place one drop of the blend on a cotton ball placed near the head)

Inability to stop worrying: rose on Yintang

Ungrounded: vetiver or spikenard on KI1

Breaking Insomnia Patterns

Some of the following suggestions can help keep the sleep cycle normal:

- No screen time 1 hour before bed.
- No stimulants, especially caffeine, at least 1 hour before bed.
- Use only soft, warm lighting at night. Try to block all light filtering into the bedroom.
- Set a regular bedtime and stick to it, even if sleep does not come. Rest or meditate, or consider visualizations of relaxing and falling asleep. Counting sheep does work!
- Recite affirmations to let go of stressful thoughts that are probably leading to sleeplessness.

Best Acupressure Point for Insomnia

GB20 • Fengchi (see Gallbladder 20, page 69)

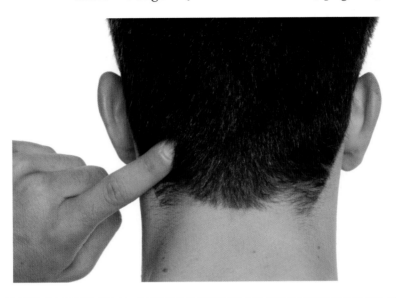

Other Acupressure Points to Consider

After pressing the best acupressure point for this condition, follow with one of these points:

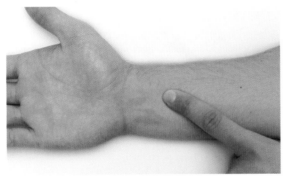

For insomnia with exhaustion, add
PC6 • Neiguan (see Pericardium 6, page 61)

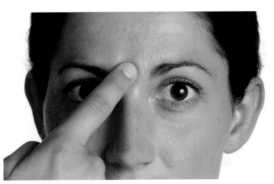

For insomnia with inability to stop
worrying, add Yintang (see page 87)

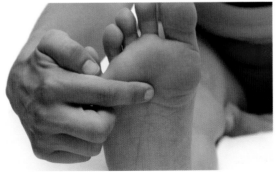

For insomnia with feeling of not
being grounded, add KI1 • Yongquan
(see Kidney 1, page 54)

Insufficient Lactation

A new mother's inability to produce enough milk to satisfy the needs of her baby may be due to mammary hypoplasia, a condition where the mammary glands in the breast tissue are insufficient. Stress can reduce milk production; ironically, this may be associated with fear of underproducing. Obesity can lead to poor glucose metabolism, suggesting insulin may be involved in the production of milk.

Signs and Symptoms

Insufficient production of milk is the main sign. Insufficient lactation may be evident in an unsatisfied need in the baby, but this can also happen with latching issues, especially if it occurs soon after birth.

Note

If the insufficiency lasts too long, it could endanger the health of the baby. Help from a lactation consultant can be very helpful, especially for new moms with first-time babies.

Other Treatments

- Herbs that improve breast milk production include goat's rue, fenugreek, alfalfa, nettles, fennel and blessed thistle
- Consider making lactation cookies (see box)

Lactation Cookies

The active ingredients in these cookies are flaxseed and brewer's yeast, which provide the necessary nutrients to increase lactation. Be sure to use brewer's yeast since other yeasts do not provide the same benefits. Recipes are available on many mothering websites.

Aromatherapy for Acupoints

Fennel on CV17

Due to exhaustion: basil on SI1

Depleted blood from delivery: Roman chamomile on SP10

Best Acupressure Point for Insufficient Lactation
CV17 • Tanzhong (see Conception Vessel 17, page 81)

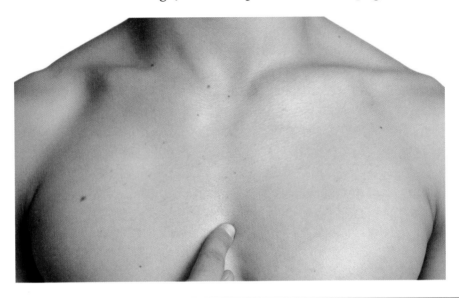

Other Acupressure Points to Consider

After pressing the best acupressure point for this condition, follow with one of these points:

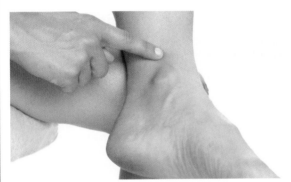

Also add SP6 • Sanyinjiao
(see Spleen 6, page 43)

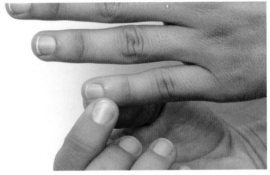

For insufficient lactation due to exhaustion,
add SI1 • Shaoze (see Small Intestine 1,
page 47)

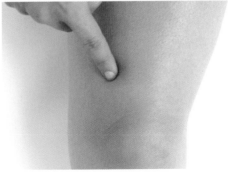

For insufficient lactation due to
blood deficiency, add SP10 • Xuehai
(see Spleen 10, page 45)

Irregular Menstruation

Irregular menstruation describes a menstrual cycle that is not proceeding on its established normal rhythm. As every woman may have a different "normal," the definition includes these unique variations. Irregularities are most commonly triggered by hormonal shifts but may be due to changes in nutritional status, increased exercise, injury or stress. Some illnesses are known to influence the cycle; specifically, polycystic ovary syndrome, pelvic inflammatory disease and fibroids all lead to changes. Irregularity may be idiopathic (unknown cause). Some medications may affect the cycle, while pregnancy will stop the cycle altogether.

Signs and Symptoms

Typical cycles are between 21 and 35 days apart. At menarche (the onset of menstruation), there may be fluctuations in many aspects of the cycle as the body adjusts to the changes in hormonal levels. Another time of natural change is perimenopause, the time around the onset of menopause (menopause is defined as 365 days since the last period. On the 366th day, the status is defined as post-menopause).

The irregularity of the rhythm may be associated with the length of time between cycles of bleeding or the number of days on which bleeding occurs. It may indicate a change in flow, either more or less volume, or breakout bleeding between cycles. Finally, it may manifest as a change of symptoms, such as increased pain or mood swings.

> ## Note
> A sudden or dramatic change could indicate a more serious condition and should be diagnosed as soon as possible. Ectopic pregnancies will stop a cycle and can be quite dangerous. The irregularity could also be due to a tumor.

Other Treatments

- Magnesium, evening primrose oil, vitamin A, vitamin C, nettles, danggui, vitex or red clover can be helpful
- Ginger tea to relax uterine spasm
- Cinnamon, iron-rich foods and B vitamins to treat excessive bleeding

Aromatherapy for Acupoints

Cypress for SP10

With cold: rosemary on LR3

Deficient or insufficient menses: helichrysum on CV3

Excess bleeding: clary sage or geranium on LR2

Cramping and pain: tarragon or clary sage on SP8

Best Acupressure Point for Irregular Menstruation

SP10 • Xuehai (see Spleen 10, page 45)

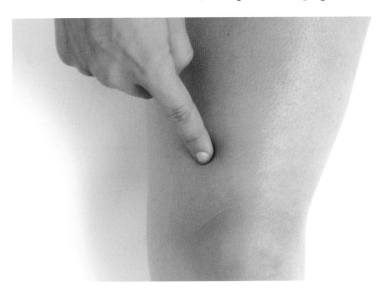

Other Acupressure Points to Consider

After pressing the best acupressure point for this condition, follow with one of these points:

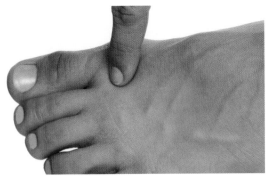

Also add LR3 • Taichong
(see Liver 3, page 74)

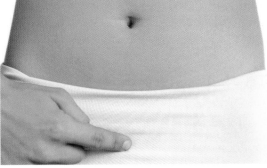

For deficient menstruation, add
CV3 • Zhongji (see Conception Vessel 3,
page 77)

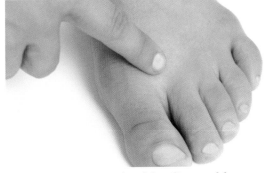

For excessive bleeding, add
LR2 • Xingjian (see Liver 2, page 73)

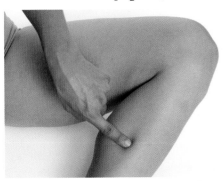

For irregular menstruation with cramping
and pain, add SP8 • Diji (see Spleen 8,
page 44)

Leukorrhea (Vaginal Discharge)

Leukorrhea is vaginal discharge. It is usually white, although it may appear yellowish. The discharge is mostly mucus and may contain pus or blood. It may occur regularly or appear suddenly. Hormonal imbalance is commonly the cause, but it may be an indication of another condition, such as a bacterial or fungal vaginal infection.

Sexual intercourse with a new partner may lead to infection as the vaginal flora adjust to the bacterial profile of the new partner. So-called honeymooner's disease is usually cystitis (urinary tract infection) but may manifest as a vaginal infection as well.

Signs and Symptoms

The term "leukorrhea" describes a primary symptom — vaginal discharge. It may be thin to thick, copious or scant, white to yellow. Red-tinged or green discharge is a sign of a more serious condition, especially if the color darkens or it is accompanied by a foul odor. Itching, pain, redness and swelling are common symptoms of a vaginal infection. Although primarily associated with sexually transmitted diseases, odor may occur with all vaginal infections.

Note

Leukorrhea may be a sign of an underlying infection. All infections should be speedily addressed, but because many sexually transmitted diseases have serious consequences, they should be treated as soon as possible.

Other Treatments

- Douche made with apple cider vinegar, tea tree oil and lecithin (see box)
- For yeast infection: plain whole milk yogurt and geranium essential oil as a vaginal pack
- Oregano oil caps

Vaginal Infection Douche

Add ¼ cup (60 mL) of apple cider vinegar to 2 cups (500 mL) of warm water. Add 5 drops of tea tree oil and a pinch of non-soy lecithin (the lecithin helps keep the oil suspended in the base). Shake well and add to a douche bag or bottle for application. May be repeated up to three times a day. See a doctor if there is no improvement after 3 days.

Aromatherapy for Acupoints

Essential oils are extremely effective at clearing bacterial infections.

Sandalwood on LR8

With pain: pain blend (see page 136) on LR2

Due to yeast: clary sage on SP8

With vaginal prolapse: rose on SP10

Best Acupressure Point for Leukorrhea
LR8 • Ququan (see Liver 8, page 75)

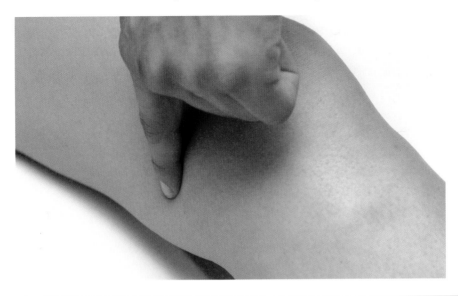

Other Acupressure Points to Consider

After pressing the best acupressure point for this condition, follow with one of these points:

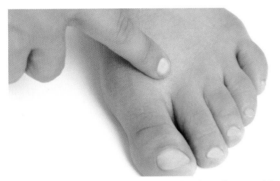

For vaginal infections and leukorrhea with pain, add LR2 • Xingjian (see Liver 2, page 73)

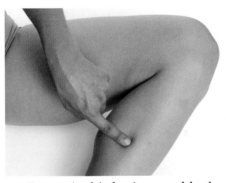

For vaginal infections and leukorrhea due to yeast, add SP8 • Diji (see Spleen 8, page 44)

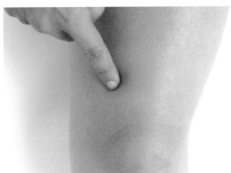

For vaginal infections and leukorrhea with vaginal prolapse, add SP10 • Xuehai (see Spleen 10, page 45)

Low Back Pain

Low back pain describes pain located in the area of the back below the ribs and may include the sacrum. Like all musculoskeletal pain, it may have many causes, but typically it arises from injury, overuse and lack of strength in the core or age. Many different muscle groups exist in the low back and any or all may be involved.

Signs and Symptoms

The pain may be aching, pulling, shooting, stabbing or throbbing; basically any kind of pain can occur in the low back. The pain may be mild to severe and intense. The problem may originate in the spine or the muscles. Muscle groups commonly involved include flexors (pain with lifting), extensors (pain bending over) or obliques (pain with twisting). Often a change in posture will relieve the pain — many who suffer from low back pain adopt a forward-leaning stance to avoid engaging the pain.

The pain may also refer to other parts of the body or be referred from internal organs. Low back pain may not originate in the back and may indicate a problem like kidney stones, uterine fibroids, endometriosis, stomach ulcers or tumors that may be at the root of it.

> ### Note
> Do not let low back pain go undiagnosed.

Other Treatments

- Eat black sesame seeds, molasses, seaweed, shellfish — all of which are high in minerals that tone and strengthen back muscles
- A few drops of tincture of lobelia applied topically can ease spasm

Juniper Berry Massage Oil

Add 3 drops of Juniper essential oil to 1 teaspoon (5 mL) of St. John's wort infused oil and massage over area of pain.

Aromatherapy for Acupoints

Clary sage on BL40

Pain blend (see page 136) on any recommended acupressure point on the next page

Best Acupressure Point for Low Back Pain

BL40 • Weizhong (see Bladder 40, page 52)

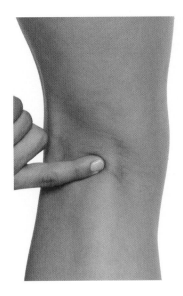

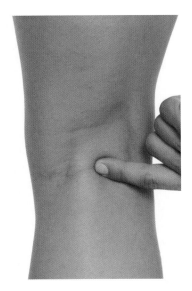

Other Acupressure Points to Consider

After pressing the best acupressure point for this condition, follow with one of these points:

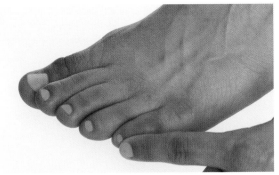

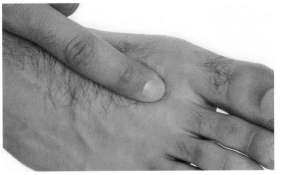

For low back pain in the sacral region, add
BL67 • Zhiyin (see Bladder 67, page 53)

For low back pain when lifting or bending,
add LR2 • Xingjian (see Liver 2, page 73)

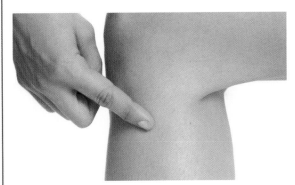

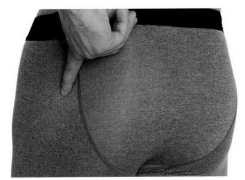

For low back pain when twisting, add
GB34 • Yanglingquan (see Gallbladder 34,
page 71)

For low back pain that radiates
down the leg, add GB30 • Huantiao
(see Gallbladder 30, page 70)

Mastitis, Breast Distention, Clogged Milk Ducts

Mastitis (inflammation of the breast tissue), breast distention and clogged milk ducts are common in postpartum moms, and any of these conditions may impede proper breastfeeding. In any of these cases, the cause may be an infection, or the baby may have poor latching technique.

Breast distention apart from pregnancy can happen as a symptom of PMS (premenstrual syndrome) and is directly related to the shift of hormones that trigger the bleeding phase of the menstrual cycle.

Signs and Symptoms

Swelling of the breast tissue is the primary symptom. There is often discomfort or pain. If there is an infection, there may be typical associated signs: redness, heat, tenderness. It is also possible to have discharge of pus from the nipple.

Note

Any infection should be addressed immediately. If the symptoms do not improve or get worse, seek medical attention.

Other Treatments

- Keep nursing or pumping. Without this, the inflammation will take much longer to resolve. The baby is perfectly equipped to digest any inflammatory compounds in the milk

Cabbage Poultice

Cabbage leaves have a long history of use to treat ailments. In fact, cabbage was mentioned in the Egyptian and Greek texts as a healing agent. Cabbage is very high in healing compounds such as vitamin C, vitamin K and lactic acid (the same compound that ferments cabbage so beautifully into sauerkraut) and is antimicrobial and diuretic, which greatly helps to reduce the inflammation and heat of mastitis.

Heat a cabbage leaf until it softens slightly and is a comfortably warm temperature. Apply the leaf over breast and leave until it cools. This can be done several times until the pain and swelling are reduced.

Aromatherapy for Acupoints

Breast distention or clogged milk ducts: lavender on SI1

Mastitis: tea tree on SI1

Breast distention or mastitis with cold sensation: ginger on ST43

Mastitis with radiating pain: rose or helichrysum on Ht7

Best Acupressure Point for Mastitis, Breast Distention, Clogged Milk Ducts

SI1 • Shaoze (see Small Intestine 1, page 47)

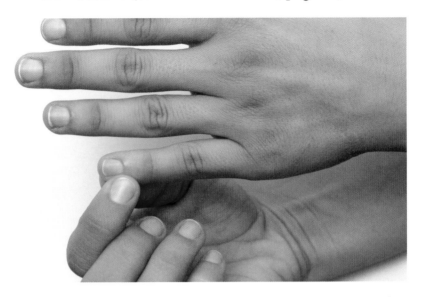

Other Acupressure Points to Consider

After pressing the best acupressure point for this condition, follow with one of these points:

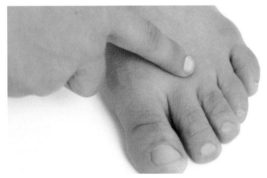

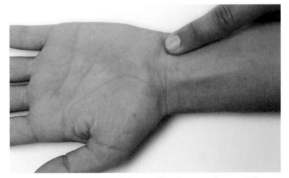

For mastitis with a cold sensation, add ST43 • Xiangu (see Stomach 43, page 41)

For mastitis with radiating pain, add Ht7 • Shenmen (see Heart 7, page 46)

Menopausal Symptoms

Hot flashes — the sensation of heat, commonly moving in a wave over the body — is the symptom most associated with the hormonal changes of menopause. Stress, spicy food, caffeine, smoking and alcohol have all been shown to worsen hot flashes. Women who exercise regularly tend to experience hot flashes less often and less severely than sedentary women.

Signs and Symptoms

In addition to the heat, there may be dizziness and a prickling sensation on the skin. Sweating is common, especially at night; in severe cases, the sheets may have to be changed several times in one night.

Post-menopausal women often experience another symptom — vaginal dryness. In fact, dryness can manifest in many ways, including skin, hair and eyes. Some women report a decreased interest in sexual activity, due in part to the discomfort from dryness. Urinary incontinence is common, and may be accompanied by increased urgency and frequency.

Other Treatments

- For vaginal dryness, use douches with lubricating herbs, such as marshmallow, slippery elm or the water used to soak flaxseeds
- Be sure to use healing oils, such as flaxseed, borage seed or evening primrose seed usually found in gelcap form. Evening primrose oil has shown good results for helping with hormonal imbalances. Borage or black currant seed oil are other options
- Seeds like flax, pumpkin or black sesame are high in minerals and strengthen the body
- Herbs to reduce symptoms, either in caps or as tea, include chaste tree, donggui and red clover
- Avoid using soap to clean the vaginal tissue. If concerned about cleanliness, consider using herbal teas as a topical rinse. Jasmine tea is wonderful for this

Aromatherapy for Acupoints

Emotional flux: rose geranium on SP6

Hot flashes: clary sage on KI6

Urinary incontinence: carrot seed on CV4

Vaginal dryness: frankincense or rose on CV1

Increasing Libido with Lubricants

Blend sandalwood, frankincense and rose essential oils with a lubricating base of aloe or the water saved from soaking flaxseeds. Consider blending in wild yam powder. Some women like to add a tiny amount of cinnamon essential oil because it is warming and stimulating (limit to only 1 drop per $\frac{1}{4}$ cup/60 mL base). Plan for extra time for foreplay.

Best Acupressure Point for Menopausal Symptoms

KI6 • Zhaohai (see Kidney 6, page 56)

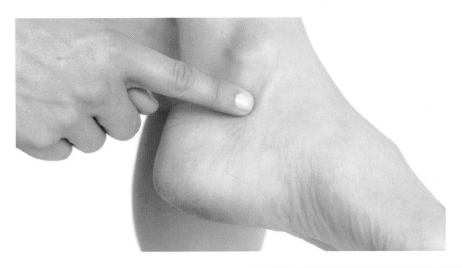

Other Acupressure Points to Consider

After pressing the best acupressure point for this condition, follow with one of these points:

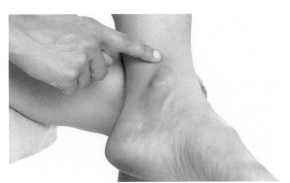

Also add SP6 • Sanyinjiao
(see Spleen 6, page 43)

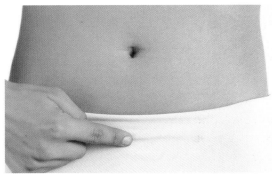

For menopausal symptoms with urinary
incontinence, add CV4 • Guanyuan
(see Conception Vessel 4, page 78)

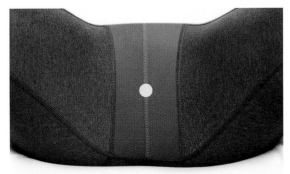

For menopausal symptoms with vaginal
dryness, add CV1 • Huiyin (see Conception
Vessel 1, page 76)

Morning Sickness

Morning sickness is an increase in nausea during pregnancy and is especially common in the first trimester, starting around week 6 and often over by week 12. It is caused by the radical shift in hormones that characterize pregnancy.

Signs and Symptoms

The nausea is usually accompanied by vomiting, which often relieves the nausea. There may be accompanying symptoms of headache, dizziness, fatigue or sweating.

A variant of this condition is referred to as hyperemesis gravidarum, which is a much more serious condition. It involves constant and unrelenting nausea and the inability to keep anything, often even water, in the system. It can lead to dehydration and electrolyte imbalances — very alarming symptoms any time, but especially when pregnant. Moms experiencing hyperemesis gravidarum often require hospitalization and intravenous nutrients and fluids.

Aromatherapy for Acupoints

Ginger or peppermint on PC6

With headache: lavender and peppermint on ST8

With weakness: black spruce on SP6

With sweating: blue chamomile on LI11

Note

The protocols outlined here may help prevent or lessen morning sickness but are not appropriate for the much more serious hyperemesis gravidarum.

Other Treatments

- Ginger tea (see box)
- Peppermint or ginger essential oil. Whichever scent appeals should be kept at bedside and sniffed immediately upon awakening. As some disorientation may occur, it is best to sniff the oil before lifting the head off the pillow

Ginger Tea Relief

Many women respond very well to ginger tea. In fact, ginger has been shown not only to be extremely safe during pregnancy, but it may also help moms with a history of miscarriage — studies have shown that ginger helps decrease uterine spasm. Add about an inch (2.5 cm) of fresh ginger root, sliced, to 1 cup (250 mL) and pour very hot but not boiling water over it. Cover and let steep for 10 to 15 minutes. Strain and enjoy.

Best Acupressure Point for Morning Sickness

PC6 • Neiguan (see Pericardium 6, page 61)

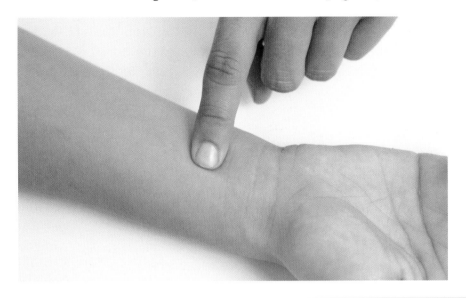

Other Acupressure Points to Consider

After pressing the best acupressure point for this condition, follow with one of these points:

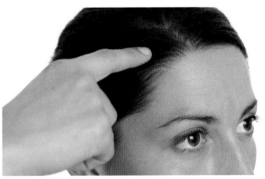

For morning sickness with headache, add
ST8 • Touwei (see Stomach 8, page 36)

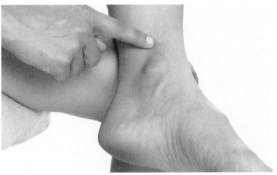

For morning sickness with weakness, add
SP6 • Sanyinjiao (see Spleen 6, page 43)

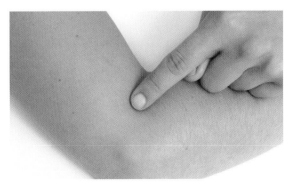

For morning sickness with sweating, add
LI11 • Quchi (see Large Intestine 11,
page 31)

Nausea and Vomiting

Nausea is a sensation often resulting in a need to vomit. Vomiting is the body's technique for removing matter from the upper gastrointestinal tract very quickly. It may result from ingesting bad food or allergens, overeating or overindulging in alcohol. Due to motion sickness, some people experience both when traveling.

Signs and Symptoms

Nausea leads to a queasy, unsettled feeling in the abdomen. There may be sweating, shaking, dizziness or fatigue. Increased salivation and activation of the gag reflex often precede the act of vomiting. Vomiting can result in sore throat, irritation and burning as stomach acid comes into prolonged contact with the tissues of the throat and mouth. Violent or extended vomiting can cause many problems as the act dramatically increases pressure in the abdomen. Some cases of prolapse, for example, can be traced to severe bouts of vomiting.

Rapid onset violent vomiting is a common sign of food poisoning. It may also signal trauma to the head, heart or digestive system. It may indicate internal bleeding, especially if there is blood in the vomit. Many patients with appendicitis experience nausea and vomiting as symptoms.

Bulimia, a disease characterized by repeated, self-induced vomiting, can deteriorate the teeth as stomach acid destroys the enamel.

Note
If vomiting is excessive or ongoing, it commonly leads to dehydration requiring hospitalization for IV fluids.

Other Treatments

- Consume enzymes with meals. Probiotics, kefir or other cultured foods can help
- Avoid eating foods that are too rich or contain complex combinations
- If nausea and vomiting is due to rancid food, clay or charcoal capsules can help absorb the irritant and ease symptoms

Slow-breathing Tip
Always take three deep, slow, relaxing breaths before eating. This activates the parasympathetic state (also called "rest and digest").

Aromatherapy for Acupoints

Ginger-peppermint on PC6

With food stagnation: ginger on CV12

With shooting pain: chamomile on ST43

With burping and indigestion: fennel on SP4

Best Acupressure Point for Nausea and Vomiting

PC6 • Neiguan (see Pericardium 6, page 61)

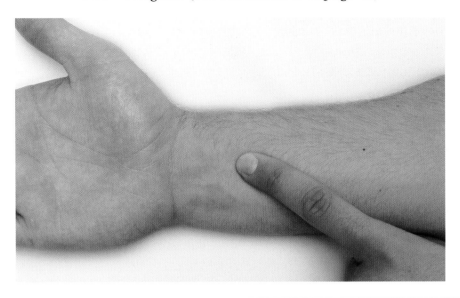

Other Acupressure Points to Consider

After pressing the best acupressure point for this condition, follow with one of these points:

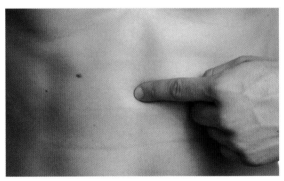

For nausea and vomiting with food stagnation, add CV12 • Zhongwan (see Conception Vessel 12, page 80)

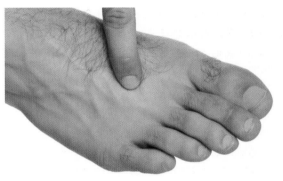

For nausea and vomiting with shooting pain, add ST43 • Xiangu (see Stomach 43, page 41)

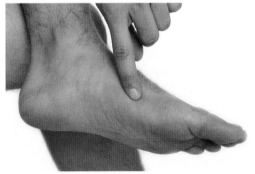

For nausea and vomiting with burping and indigestion, add SP4 • Gongsun (see Spleen 4, page 42)

Nocturnal Enuresis (Bedwetting)

Bedwetting is common in children, especially as they transition from diapers to using a toilet. Potty training takes some time as the child learns to have control over their urinary system. Nighttime, of course, is the most difficult time. At times, bedwetting will continue past the toddler stage, and in some children (and adults) there may be episodes due to infection or bladder disease. Emotional or psychological reasons may also be involved; for example, nightmares can lead to bedwetting.

Signs and Symptoms

Wetting the bed, obviously, is the main sign of the inability to control the bladder at night. There may be pain and discharge if an infection is the cause. There is often anguish, dishonesty or fear from the child, as they feel distress over the condition.

Extended bedwetting well past the conventional age of potty training, or secondary bedwetting — when the behavior returns after control has been established — may be indicators that the situation needs more attention.

Other Treatments

- Avoid beverages near bedtime. Urinate at the same time right before bed
- Avoid diuretic foods, such as celery, cucumbers, lettuce, beets and most fruit (as well as foods containing caffeine), close to bedtime
- Start the practice of qigong early! The first lesson concentrates on a clear understanding of the body's boundaries and includes movements that strengthen the perineum
- Kegel exercises to strengthen muscles
- Intentionally stopping the urine stream mid-flow can help reprogram the nerves and muscles that govern the sphincters
- Oregano capsules may help

Aromatherapy for Acupoints

Cypress on SP6

Cinnamon on GV20

Copious and frequent episodes: rosemary on KI6

Due to infection: thyme on CV1

Preventive Bedwetting Drink

To prepare, mix 1 teaspoon (5 mL) of apple cider vinegar, 1/2 teaspoon (2 mL) of raw honey (only use for children over 1 year) and a pinch of cinnamon into a small glass of water. Take after dinner but at least 2 hours before bedtime.

Best Acupressure Point for Nocturnal Enuresis

SP6 • Sanyinjiao (see Spleen 6, page 43)

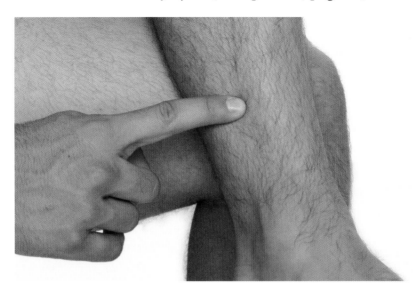

Other Acupressure Points to Consider

After pressing the best acupressure point for this condition, follow with one of these points:

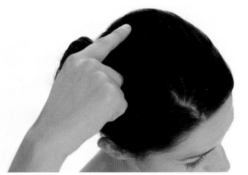

For nocturnal enuresis due to bladder prolapse, add GV20 • Baihui (see Governing Vessel 20, page 84)

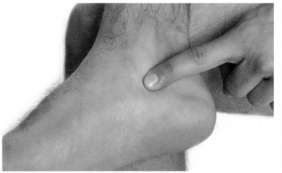

For nocturnal enuresis with copious and frequent episodes, add KI6 • Zhaohai (see Kidney 6, page 56)

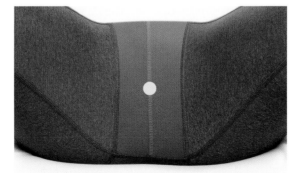

For nocturnal enuresis with bladder infection, add CV1 • Huiyin (see Conception Vessel 1, page 76)

Phlegm

Phlegm is another name for mucus, the substance that lines the mucous membranes of the body, especially those of the gastrointestinal and respiratory systems. The function of mucus is to moisturize and lubricate the tissues where it is found; this is usually the work of thinner mucus secretions. Sticky mucus will catch and hold irritants, stopping them from proceeding further down the respiratory tract. Finally, mucus contains its own immune factors, substances like antibodies and enzymes, that recognize pathogens and tag them for removal or break them down at the site.

The term "phlegm" is mostly used to describe the thickened mucus that is difficult to expel. In the respiratory tract, mucus usually leads to increased expectoration as the lungs work to cough it out. In the digestive tract, mucus that dries out and thickens can lead to increased symptoms of constipation.

Signs and Symptoms

The main sign is excess, thickened mucus in the respiratory system, with an increased tendency to cough. Phlegm is most commonly seen in the digestive system when an enema or colonic is used, as the water removes stuck phlegm from the colon.

If the phlegm is very stubborn, the body's attempts to expel it may cause injuries. Coughing, for example, may lead to a sore throat or, in extreme cases, prolapse of organs such as the bladder or uterus as the increase in pressure bears down and weakens the connective tissues.

Other Treatments

- Use steams with the recommended essential oils (see box)
- Apply chest rub with peppermint, pine, fir and/or spruce (see page 170)
- Cupped-hand tapotement massage (rhythmic tapping) on the upper back helps clear mucus
- Avoiding dairy may lessen phlegm production, although raw milk is known as a remedy to reduce phlegm

Aromatherapy for Acupoints

Juniper on ST40

For digestive phlegm: ginger or black pepper on SP4

For excessive respiratory phlegm: eucalyptus globulus on LU11

With lack of energy to cough: Hyssop var. decumbens or spruce on LU7

Steam Inhalation for Phlegm

To prepare a steam inhalation, bring a pot of water to a boil, then allow it to cool to a breathable temperature — test it before adding oils. Add 1 drop each of eucalyptus globulus and spruce essential oils. Be sure to start cautiously by sniffing it without a head towel first, then cover the head with a towel to catch the steam and inhale for several minutes.

Best Acupressure Point for Phlegm

ST40 • Fenglong (see Stomach 40, page 40)

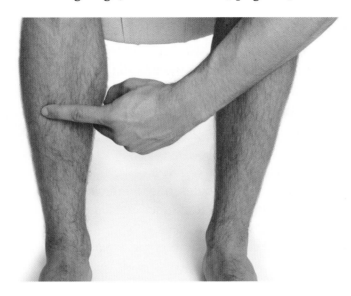

Other Acupressure Points to Consider

After pressing the best acupressure point for this condition, follow with one of these points:

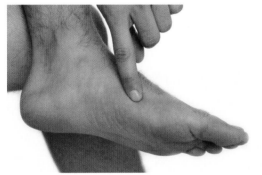

For digestive phlegm (phlegm in the stool), add SP4 • Gongsun (see Spleen 4, page 42)

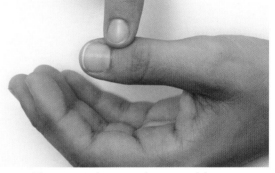

For excessive respiratory phlegm production, add LU11 • Shaoshang (see Lung 11, page 28)

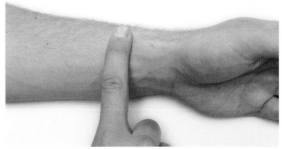

For respiratory phlegm with lack of energy to cough, add LU7 • Lieque (see Lung 7, page 25)

Plantar Fasciitis

Plantar fasciitis is used to describe inflammation of the plantar fascia, the connective tissue that forms the arch of the foot as it connects the toes to the heel. The act of walking depends a great deal on this band of tissue. Wearing ill-fitting shoes, jogging, or simply walking more than usual can cause plantar fasciitis. The condition can also arise after weight gain, and may be experienced during pregnancy. Foot abnormalities may also be involved, such as the tendency to roll in (pronate) or out (supinate) on the foot when walking. Long-term standing on hard surfaces may also lead to arch problems.

Signs and Symptoms

Pain and stiffness of the arch are the main symptoms. Typically, the symptoms are worse after rest but may also be aggravated with increased use. There may be weakness that extends up the calf.

> ### Note
> It is important to get a differential diagnosis to rule out arthritis or other conditions.

Other Treatments

• Consider new shoes, especially sports shoes. Avoid uncomfortable or too-small shoes

Deep Massage

Massage is very important for healing plantar fasciitis. Rolling the foot over a tennis ball is helpful for many, or try a foot roller massage tool. In the acute stage, it may be too painful to do much stretching, but attempt to stretch the fascia as soon and as often as possible, massaging in pain blend (see page 136) or one of the single essential oils listed above, deeply kneading the tissue as tolerated. If it is a long-term chronic case, it is important to focus the massage on the calf muscles first, as they tend to compensate for the lack of function.

Aromatherapy for Acupoints

Rosemary or lemongrass on KI1

Pain blend (see page 136) on any of the acupressure points on the next page

Due to pronation: bay laurel on SP4

With foot and calf weakness: helichrysum on LR3

Best Acupressure Point for Plantar Fasciitis

KI1 • Yongquan (see Kidney 1, page 54)

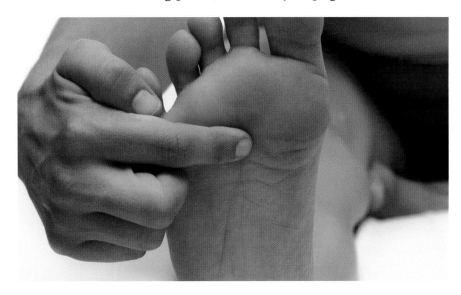

Other Acupressure Points to Consider

After pressing the best acupressure point for this condition, follow with one of these points:

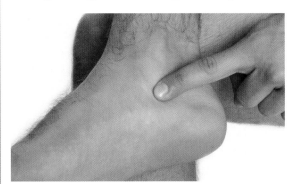

Also add KI6 • Zhaohai
(see Kidney 6, page 56)

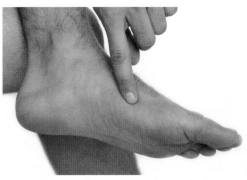

For plantar fasciitis with medial pain due
to pronation, add SP4 • Gongsun
(see Spleen 4, page 42)

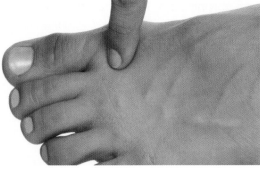

For plantar fasciitis with foot and calf
weakness, add LR3 • Taichong (see Liver 3,
page 74)

Prostatitis

Prostatitis is an inflammation of the prostate gland that may be caused by infection (acute or chronic bacterial prostatitis) or not (inflammatory prostatitis). Inflammatory prostatitis (also called non-bacterial variant) is another term for a chronically enlarged prostate gland. It may be acute, especially if caused by a recent surgery that required a catheter. Anal sex may lead to inflammation or infection if the tissue is torn.

Signs and Symptoms

The most commonly reported symptom is more frequent urination, with greater urgency but reduced output. Urination may also cause pain that may refer to areas served by the hypogastric and pelvic nerves, the nerves that govern the prostate. Because the branches of these nerves are responsible for some aspects of sexual activity, there may also be erectile dysfunction. There may also be reduced bowel function. If the condition is caused by infection, symptoms such as body aches, fever, chills and fatigue may be present.

Note
If any symptoms of infection are present (see above), see a doctor. If symptoms have not improved by the suggestions here, they may be a sign of a more serious situation. Seek medical attention.

Other Treatments
- Use a rectal suppository (see box)
- Try oregano capsules for infectious prostatitis
- Useful supplements include saw palmetto capsules, nettle root capsules, vitamin E and selenium
- Consume pumpkin seeds, Brazil nuts and turmeric

Aromatherapy for Acupoints

Oregano on CV1

With pain: geranium on LR2

Reduced urinary output: cypress on LR8

With general weakness: ginger on CV4

Difficult urination and defecation: peppermint on ST40

Rectal Suppository

To prepare a homemade rectal suppository, melt 1 tablespoon (15 mL) of coconut oil and 1 teaspoon (5 mL) of cocoa butter or shea butter until liquid. Remove from heat and add 25 drops of caullophyllum fixed oil. Allow to cool until it starts to thicken, then add 2 drops of oregano oil and 4 drops each of lavender and rosemary essential oils. Refrigerate until nearly solid, then quickly shape the substance into a long roll about the diameter of a pencil. Break roll into thumb-sized pieces and wrap in waxed paper. Store in the refrigerator. Insert one into the rectum before bed. Line underpants with a thin washcloth. If there is no change in symptoms after a week, discontinue and consult a doctor.

Best Acupressure Point for Prostatitis

CV1 • Huiyin (see Conception Vessel 1, page 76)

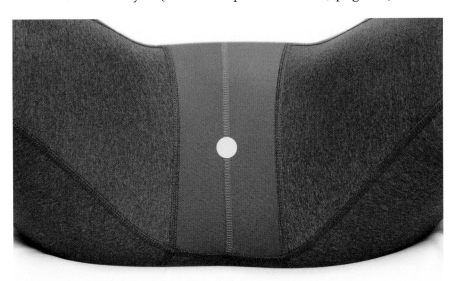

Other Acupressure Points to Consider

After pressing the best acupressure point for this condition, follow with one of these points:

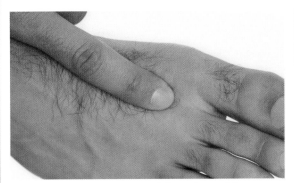

For prostatitis with pain, add
LR2 • Xingjian (see Liver 2, page 73)

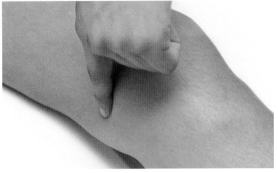

For prostatitis with leakage, add
LR8 • Ququan (see Liver 8, page 75)

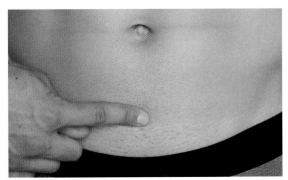

For prostatitis with general weakness, add
CV4 • Guanyuan (see Conception Vessel 4,
page 78)

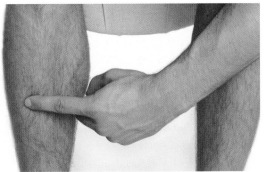

For prostatitis with edema, add
ST40 • Fenglong (see Stomach 40,
page 40)

Raynaud Syndrome

Raynaud syndrome is an inappropriate narrowing of blood vessels in the hands and the feet, especially when the digits become cold or the affected person experiences stress. The condition affects the thumb, first and second fingers and part of the third finger. These digits are specifically affected because the hand and fingers are served by two different arteries, the radial artery and the ulnar artery. The condition can happen in the lower leg and feet as well.

Signs and Symptoms

The main symptoms reflect the impeded blood flow — the hands or feet may become very pale, bluish or red as the blood flow changes. There may be tingling, numbness and reduced function. Pain usually happens when the blood flow returns to the area.

The syndrome is much more common in women. It has been suggested that it could result from a buildup of toxic substances in the body because the condition is found more commonly among people who work with certain chemicals, such as those found in the plastics manufacturing industry. Repetitive motions, especially those that involve vibrations, such as playing the piano, may increase the likelihood of developing this syndrome.

Other Treatments

- Pain blend (see page 136) can help with moving the blood, while Roman chamomile may relax the spasm of the blood vessels
- Consider capsaicin cream for extreme cold and pale hands
- Take a warm (not hot) water bath with Epsom salts

Aromatherapy for Acupoints

Helichrysum on LU9

Due to age or debility: rosemary on KI3

With red burning: Roman chamomile on LU7

With blood deficiency: rose on Ht7

Best Acupressure Point for Raynaud Syndrome

LU9 • Taiyuan (see Lung 9, page 26)

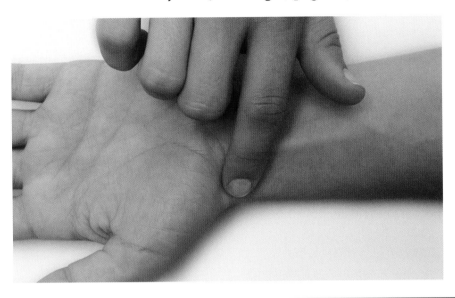

Other Acupressure Points to Consider

After pressing the best acupressure point for this condition, follow with one of these points:

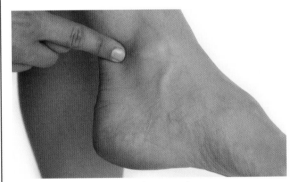

For Raynaud syndrome due to age or debility, add KI3 • Taixi (see Kidney 3, page 55)

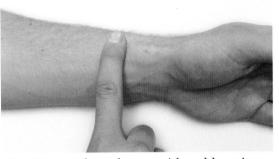

For Raynaud syndrome with red burning, add LU7 • Lieque (see Lung 7, page 25)

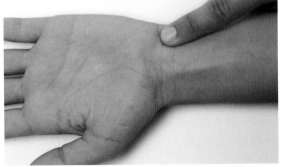

For Raynaud syndrome with blood deficiency, add Ht7 • Shenmen (see Heart 7, page 46)

Rhinitis (Runny or Stuffy Nose)

A stuffy nose and a runny nose both result from inflammation of the nasal passages. A stuffy or runny nose is a common sign of many different conditions, including a cold, flu, allergies and sinus infection, which all commonly lead to drainage symptoms. Inhaling an irritant will stimulate this natural defense, which works to remove the irritant. Spicy food, for example, is a well-known "irritant."

Signs and Symptoms

With a stuffy nose, the inflammation is so great it is restricting the flow of mucus, whereas with a runny nose, the increased secretions are more obvious. Typically, secretions are clear, watery and copious. Tearing of the eyes is a common accompanying symptom. There may be pain, especially if the pressure builds in the sinus cavities because of inflammation. An often overlooked symptom is foggy brain, as the immune response overwhelms our ability to function clearly. If a runny nose continues long enough, it can lead to irritation of the tissues, both in the nose and below it, as well as on the nostrils.

If the mucus changes in color or becomes dark, it is usually a sign of infection. Bleeding may be a sign of irritated tissue or a more serious problem.

Other Treatments

- For thin clear secretions: warming oil like black pepper or ginger can be used as a steam (see page 226 for directions). Be sure to keep the eyes closed at all times if you're using steam
- For thick-colored secretions: inula (a mucolytic essential oil), eucalyptus, peppermint and/or Hyssopus var. decumbens (these can also be used as a steam; see above)
- Steam with blue chamomile. Chamomile tea bags, warm (not hot) over eyes for tearing
- Nettles as a food year-round; foods rich in quercitin (or capsules)

Aromatherapy for Acupoints

Runny nose: sage on LI20

With tearing eyes: blue chamomile on BL2

With frontal headache or pain: rosemary on GB14

With constant draining: holy basil on GV20

Nasal Wash

Cleansing the sinuses with a neti pot, nasal syringe or nasal spray may help. To prepare the formula to treat thin clear secretions, add ½ teaspoon (2 mL) of apple cider vinegar to ½ cup (125 mL) of warm water and add it to the device. For thick secretions, add ¼ teaspoon (1 mL) of salt to ½ cup (125 mL) of warm water and add to the device. Follow the directions for the device used.

Best Acupressure Point for Rhinitis

LI20 • Yingxiang (see Large Intestine 20, page 33)

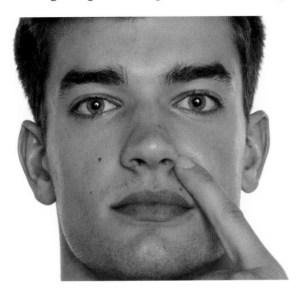

Other Acupressure Points to Consider

After pressing the best acupressure point for this condition, follow with one of these points:

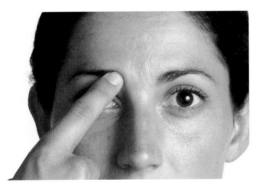

For rhinitis with tearing eyes, add
BL2 • Zanzhu (see Bladder 2, page 50)

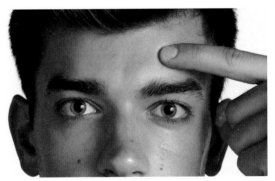

For rhinitis with frontal headache or pain,
add GB14 • Yangbai (see Gallbladder 14,
page 68)

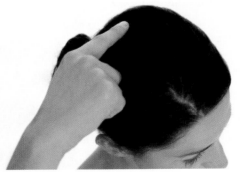

For rhinitis with constant draining, add
GV20 • Baihui (see Governing Vessel 20,
page 84)

Sciatica

As a condition, sciatica describes pain that originates deep in the posterior pelvic girdle and radiates along the sciatic nerve, which runs down the back of the leg. The pain is due to an odd anomaly of anatomy — the sciatic nerve runs between two muscles, the piriformis and obturator. If either muscle becomes inflamed, the nerve is trapped, leading to pain from the pressure. A variant, called piriformis syndrome, happens when the nerve pierces the belly of the piriformis muscle itself, resulting in a much greater likelihood of impingement. Sciatica usually occurs unilaterally (one-sided) but can happen in both legs at the same time.

Signs and Symptoms

The primary symptom is pain, especially down the back of either leg. Other symptoms include tingling and numbness, which often occurs in the "saddle" region — the buttocks and inner thighs. Shooting electric sensations, diminished reflexes and reduced function of the affected side are common. When the effects extend to the foot and function is limited, a symptom called foot drop (difficulty keeping the foot flexed) may result.

If sciatica occurs in both legs at the same time or results in incontinence, it can be a condition called cauda equina syndrome. This is a much more serious condition of inflammation of the nerve roots deep in the spine — see a doctor.

Other Treatments
- St. John's wort oil topically for its nerve regenerative properties
- St. John's wort capsules
- B vitamins, magnesium and evening primrose oil

Aromatherapy for Acupoints

Pain blend (see page 136) on GB30

With numbness: pain blend (see page 136) on KI3

With poor circulation: rosemary or helichrysum on SP10

With low back pain: basil on BL40

Best Acupressure Point for Sciatica

GB30 • Huantiao (see Gallbladder 30, page 70)

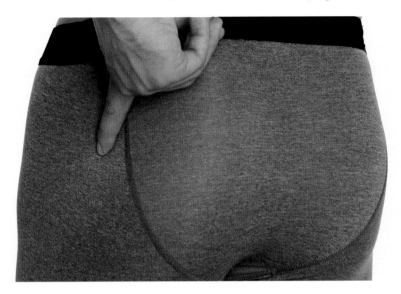

Other Acupressure Points to Consider

After pressing the best acupressure point for this condition, follow with one of these points:

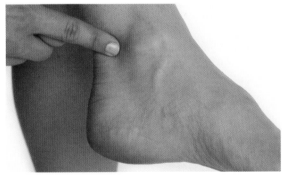

For sciatica with numbness, add
KI3 • Taixi (see Kidney 3, page 55)

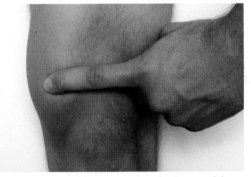

For sciatica with poor circulation, add
SP10 • Xuehai (see Spleen 10, page 45)

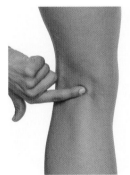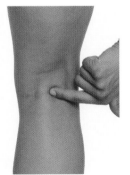

For sciatica with low back pain, add
BL40 • Weizhong (see Bladder 40, page 52)

Skin Blemishes (Acne)

Skin irritations occur when the skin is not efficiently turning over skin cells or processing sebum, resulting in clogged pores. If the site becomes infected, it becomes red and inflamed. These infections may arise because of hormonal changes, stress, changes in diet or other reasons. Skin eruptions can result from changes in beneficial bacteria that exist naturally on the skin. Ironically, overly harsh cleansing products designed specifically to eradicate blemishes may cause these changes. The following protocols may be helpful for acne rosacea as well; however, since it is an autoimmune condition, it is even more important to avoid irritating the skin and reduce stress.

Some medications may also interfere with healthy populations on the skin. Mechanical irritation, such as scrubbing the skin too vigorously or tight clothing rubbing on the skin, can also lead to eruptions. Dietary choices may increase the likelihood of developing skin problems and dietary changes may help reverse the situation. Allergies are also frequently seen to cause skin imbalances. Certain nutritional deficiencies, especially of fat-soluble vitamins like vitamin A and E, are also known to cause blemishes.

Signs and Symptoms

If the blemish is simply a clogged pore, it is called a blackhead or whitehead. If the irritation becomes infected and inflamed, usually as a result of bacterial infection, it is a pimple. Acne is a combination of all of these, and may also involve painful cysts under the skin. Skin blemishes can appear anywhere on the body, especially where nutritional deficiencies are involved. Vitamin A deficiency rash commonly appears on the posterior surface of the upper arms, and Vitamin B deficiency is the cause of pellagra.

Irritated skin should always be handled gently. What is needed in most cases is simply cleaning and treating the skin with certain oils to achieve clearer skin. Too much pressure when attempting to extract a blackhead or pimple can lead to permanent damage of the tissue and has been shown to increase the likelihood of developing acne.

Other Treatments

- Use a balancing oil blend on the face (see box)
- Vitamins A (or its precursor, beta-carotene), E, K and C from whole foods or in supplemental form may help support healthy skin
- Try silica, selenium, omega fatty acids, evening primrose or borage seed oil capsules

Aromatherapy for Acupoints

Skin balancing: patchouli or rose on ST7

Skin eruptions: rosemary verbenone on LI11

Inflammation, especially on nose: blue chamomile on LI20

Excessive oil production: cypress on Yintang and ST8

Blemish Ointment

Using a balancing oil blend on the face can help. For the base, add 15 drops of jojoba or argan oil and combine with 1 drop of blue chamomile, 1 drop of frankincense and 1 drop of rose oils. Apply regularly on blemish.

Best Acupressure Point for Skin Blemishes

ST7 • Xiaguan (see Stomach 7, page 35)

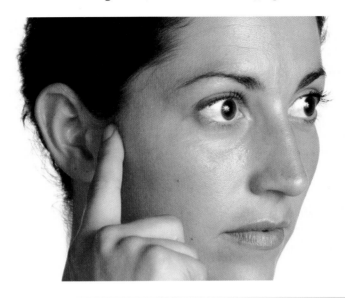

Other Acupressure Points to Consider

After pressing the best acupressure point for this condition, follow with one of these points:

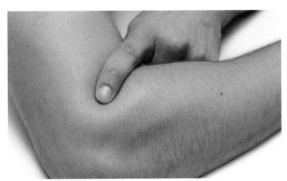

For skin eruptions, add
LI11 • Quchi (see Large Intestine 11,
page 31)

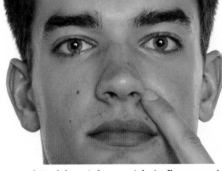

For skin blemishes with inflammation,
especially on nose, add LI20 • Yingxiang
(see Large Intestine 20, page 33)

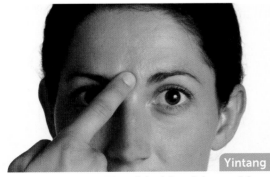

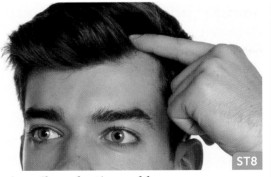

For skin blemishes with excessive oil production, add
Yintang (page 87) and ST8 • Touwei (see Stomach 8, page 36)

Sore Throat

Sore throat is most often described as a raw or irritated throat. The symptoms can appear in different locations; for example, the pharynx (pharyngitis) or larynx (laryngitis). The most common cause of sore throat is viral infection. In fact, sore throat is often the first symptom of a cold or flu.

Sore throat may also result from overuse; singers and public speakers often experience it. Inhalants and pollution can lead to throat irritation, as can post-nasal drip from a cold, allergies or sinus infection. Acid reflux at night may lead to sore throat upon rising.

Signs and Symptoms

Soreness, a raw feeling, burning, swelling and redness are all typical signs of a sore throat. The throat may itch or ache before the other symptoms appear. There may be hoarseness or total loss of voice (laryngitis). Rapid onset, swollen lymph nodes, a fever and a characteristic throat rash are usually reliable indicators to determine whether the sore throat is from a strep infection.

Most people are familiar with strep throat, also known as group A strep. Caused by the *Streptococcus pyogenes* bacteria, strep throat is quite virulent and may be dangerous if left untreated, especially in children.

Note

Some people develop an ache in the throat when fatigued. This may be linked to thyroid dysfunction and should be checked out. If strep throat is suspected or if the sore throat is accompanied by a fever over 102°F (38.9°C), see a doctor for a diagnosis.

Other Treatments

- Loss-of-voice throat sprays are prepared with herbs high in mucilage, such as marshmallow, and are easy to make at home, although there are several options at most health food stores
- Slippery elm drops (store-bought or homemade) may help
- Purslane is mucilaginous and high in omega-3 fats, which make it a great food for sore throat. Okra is another soothing vegetable

Sore Throat Soother

Add 1 drop of Ravintsara to 1 teaspoon (5 mL) of manuka honey. Allow the honey to slowly melt down the throat. The blend can be used preventively when people around us are becoming sick or at the first sign of throat irritation.

Aromatherapy for Acupoints

Due to overuse: spruce or pine on KI6

Due to virus: Ravintsara or eucalyptus on LU11

Due to allergies: blue chamomile on LI4

With strep throat: thyme on ST43

With laryngitis: Ravintsara on CV23

Best Acupressure Point for Sore Throat

KI6 • Zhaohai (see Kidney 6, page 56)

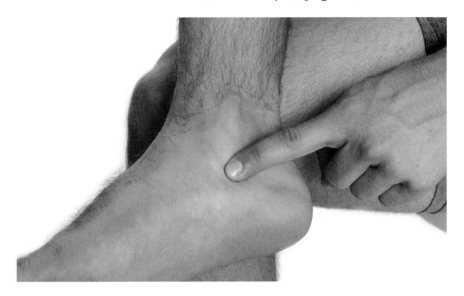

Other Acupressure Points to Consider

After pressing the best acupressure point for this condition, follow with one of these points:

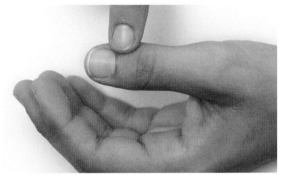

For sore throat due to virus, add
LU11 • Shaoshang (see Lung 11, page 28)

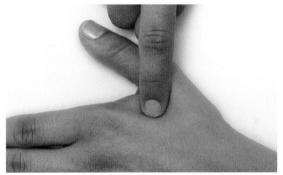

For sore throat due to allergies, add
LI4 • Hegu (see Large Intestine 4, page 29)

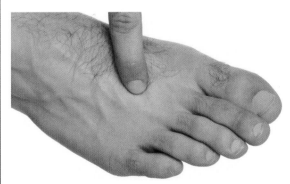

For sore throat with strep, add
ST43 • Xiangu (see Stomach 43, page 41)

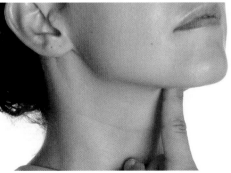

For sore throat with laryngitis, add
CV23 • Lianquan (see Conception
Vessel 23, page 83)

Thyroid Imbalance

Hypothyroidism is an underactive thyroid. Despite an abundance of thyroid-stimulating hormone circulating in the system, the gland produces less of the two main hormones, T3 and T4. There are several causes. The gland itself may be unable to function properly or the pituitary may be involved. When the immune system generates antibodies against the gland, it is called Hashimoto's disease.

Hyperthyroidism describes an overactive gland producing too much thyroid hormone. The autoimmune variant is called Grave's disease. The majority of thyroid imbalance manifests as hyperactivity of the gland.

Signs and Symptoms

Signs of hypothyroidism/Hashimoto's disease is a slowed metabolism, which leads to weight gain and, commonly, depression. Menstrual periods are heavier and longer. The eyelids swell. Typically, those with hypothyroidism are intolerant to cold. Similarly to hyperthyroidism, however, there is increased risk of atherosclerosis and heart disease.

Hyperthyroidism/Grave's disease, as might be expected, largely manifests in the opposite direction. An enlarged thyroid gland, appearing as swelling in the front of the neck over the gland (known as a goiter), is commonly seen. Exopthalmos — when pressure builds behind the eyes and presses them forward so they protrude from the sockets — may also occur. As in hypothyroidism, there is an increased risk of hypertension and heart disease. Weight loss is typical. In women, periods become lighter and shorter. Intolerance of heat, irritability and anxiety are all common symptoms.

Endocrine dysfunction is always important to detect and diagnose, as the endocrine system and the hormones it produces are responsible for so many physiological functions. The suggestions here may help the shift back to balance.

Other Treatments

- Avoid fluoride and soy products — both can lead to hormonal imbalance
- Have micronutrient levels checked, as deficiencies exacerbate thyroid issues
- Try an amino acid blend supplement
- Apply iodine to the skin, which allows it to be absorbed transdermally, to help balance the thyroid. Follow the direction on the product.
- Seaweed, especially bladderwrack, has a track record of helping with thyroid imbalances, especially if radiation — medical or environmental — is responsible for glandular dysfunction

Aromatherapy for Acupoints

Black pepper on ST9

With fatigue: spruce or pine on SP6

With weight gain: cinnamon on SP8

With weight loss: orange on CV12

Caution
Do not take iodine internally.

Best Acupressure Point for Thyroid Imbalance

ST9 • Renying (see Stomach 9, page 37)

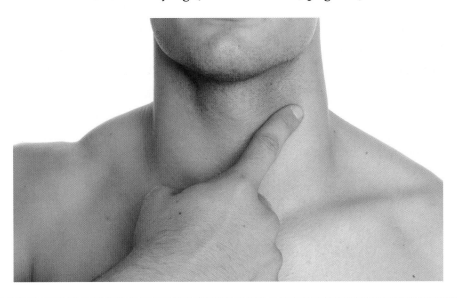

Other Acupressure Points to Consider

After pressing the best acupressure point for this condition, follow with one of these points:

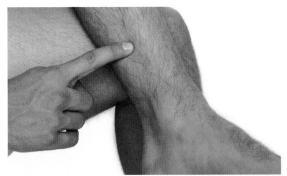

For thyroid imbalance with fatigue, add SP6 • Sanyinjiao (see Spleen 6, page 43)

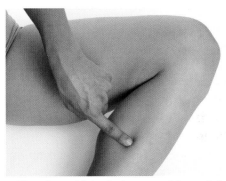

For thyroid imbalance with weight gain, add SP8 • Diji (see Spleen 8, page 44)

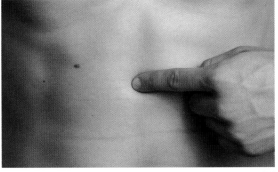

For thyroid imbalance with weight loss, add CV12 • Zhongwan (see Conception Vessel 12, page 80)

Tinnitus (Ringing in the Ears)

Tinnitus is the medical term for ringing in the ears. It may be the result of damage to the eardrums, sometimes from listening to loud music years earlier. Many musicians develop tinnitus as a result of not wearing ear protection.

Literally hundreds of pharmaceutical medications for a wide range of conditions list tinnitus as a potential side effect. A blow to the head that brings on (typically) temporary tinnitus may become permanent in some cases. Tinnitus will commonly arise in the elderly as the structures of the ear deteriorate with age. More rarely, it may develop as a result of blocked eustachian tubes. Treatments to clear the block often completely resolve the issue.

Signs and Symptoms

The condition can manifest suddenly as a high-pitched tone or slowly over many years, which usually results in a low-tone roaring sound. The sound is usually found to be very irritating and may lead to psychological issues.

Tinnitus may also be the result of certain nutritional deficiencies, such as zinc and some B vitamins in particular. Be sure to have vitamin levels tested if tinnitus develops.

Other Treatments

• Ginkgo biloba is useful where there is a known restriction of blood flow to the area, possibly from injury

Aromatherapy for Acupoints

Due to exhaustion after illness: geranium on ST36

Low-pitched and slow onset: basil on KI3

High-pitched and sudden: spikenard on LR3

Loud and constant: frankincense on GB3

Help with Acupuncture

Acupuncture has a clinical history of resolving tinnitus. Some studies show a clear reduction in symptoms after treatment. The acupressure and aromatherapy protocols described here have been beneficial both for reducing symptoms and extending the benefits of acupuncture treatments.

Best Acupressure Point For Tinnitus

ST36 • Zusanli (see Stomach 36, page 39)

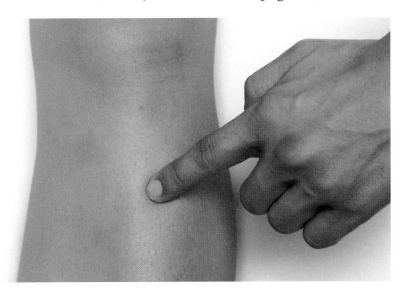

Other Acupressure Points to Consider

After pressing the best acupressure point for this condition, follow with one of these points:

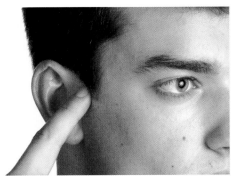

Also add GB3 • Shanguan
(see Gallbladder 3, page 66)

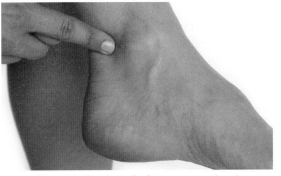

For low-pitched and slow onset tinnitus,
add KI3 • Taixi (see Kidney 3, page 55)

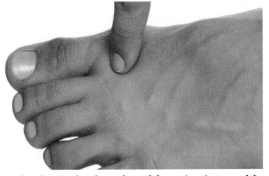

For high-pitched and sudden tinnitus, add
LR3 • Taichong (see Liver 3, page 74)

Toothache

Toothache involves damage to the tooth. It may be a symptom of tooth decay, in particular when the decay reaches the nerve of the tooth and sends a pain signal. A cracked tooth will also lead to pain. Poor circulation to the gums may lead to weak, sensitive teeth.

Signs and Symptoms

Pain is the main symptom. It may be difficult or impossible to chew with the teeth on the painful side. If the source of the problem is infection, there may be swelling and redness. It is possible to see infected discharge around the decaying tooth, usually accompanied by a foul odor.

Temporomandibular joint (TMJ) syndrome, a misalignment of the jaw due to injury or repetitive motion, often results in pain that may be difficult to distinguish from tooth decay. It is a good idea to get a diagnosis from a doctor or dentist because the conditions are treated quite differently.

Other Treatments

- Add one drop of peppermint oil to ¼ tsp (1 mL) of baking soda. Mix well. Wet the toothbrush with hydrogen peroxide and dip it into the baking soda mix. It will foam up immediately, so don't do this until you are ready to brush. Rinse well.
- Spilanthes, echinacea, myrrh and goldenseal may strengthen the gums, which affect the teeth
- CoQ10 helps the blood circulate to the tiny capillaries of the gum and reduces oxidation
- A good calcium-magnesium supplement is recommended
- Vitamin D helps heal gums, as does vitamin C

Calm Gum Infection

Oil pulling, which can be helpful in clearing old pockets of infection in the gums, is a technique from Ayurvedic medicine. It involves swishing sesame oil in your mouth for at least 20 minutes. Do not swallow! It is best to start with a few minutes and work your way up. Regular oil pulling may lead to stronger gums, which means the gums are more efficient at nourishing the teeth.

Aromatherapy for Acupoints

Myrrh on KI3

Top teeth: grapefruit on ST7, LI5

Bottom teeth: frankincense on ST6, LU10

Infection: rose on ST43

Caution

Clove oil can be used sparingly to temporarily reduce tooth pain. Do not use more than three drops a day for no more than a few days at most.

Best Acupressure Point for Toothache
KI3 • Taixi (see Kidney 3, page 55)

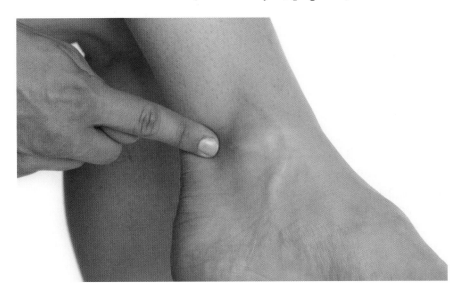

Other Acupressure Points to Consider

After pressing the best acupressure point for this condition, follow with one of these points:

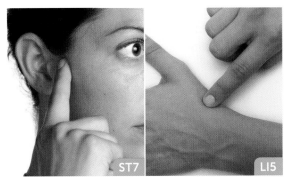

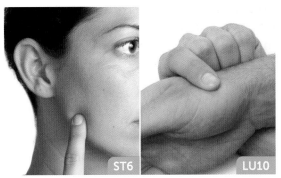

For toothache in the top teeth, add ST7 • Xiaguan (see Stomach 7, page 35) with LI5 • Yangxi (see Large Intestine 5, page 30)

For toothache in the bottom teeth, add ST6 • Jiache (Stomach 6, see page 34) with LU10 • Yuji (see Lung 10, page 27)

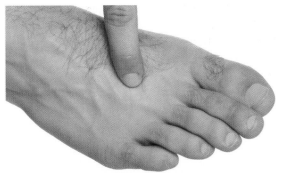

For toothache with infection, add ST43 • Xiangu (see Stomach 43, page 41)

Torticollis (Neck Spasm, Stiff Neck)

Stiff neck is an extremely common condition most people have felt at some point in their lives. It is often a result of overuse or poor posture. Sleeping positions often lead to a stiff neck upon awakening.

Torticollis is a more severe condition of stiff neck associated with muscle spasm or contraction, and is usually chronic. Torticollis may be genetic or could be due to a traumatic injury.

Signs and Symptoms

Stiff neck symptoms include muscle tension, stiffness and usually pain. It may be accompanied by headache, eye pain or shoulder pain.

Torticollis looks like an exaggerated version of the same symptoms. There is often torsion (twisting) and a dramatically reduced range of motion. In some cases, there may be tonic torticollis, which is little to no motion as the contracted muscle locks up the whole neck. On the other hand, there may be involuntary movements like shaking or twitching, known as clonic torticollis. The pain may be extreme.

Note
Torticollis may require medical intervention to relax the contracted muscle. The condition is often treated with Botox injections, which "paralyze" the muscle so that it cannot contract.

Other Treatments

- Many yoga poses focus on lengthening and strengthening the muscles of the neck
- Massage may ease stiffness and pain, but may not be well tolerated in torticollis
- Warm compresses using the pain blend (see page 136) will soften the stiffness and reduce pain
- Lobelia tincture used topically will release a spastic muscle
- Practice stress-reduction techniques. Stress locks up the neck and shoulders first

Aromatherapy for Acupoints

Ylang and geranium are antispasmodic and, once diluted, may be applied to the origin of the spasm.

Pain and stiffness: Pain blend (see page 136) on neck where pain occurs.

Stretching the Neck

It is imperative that the muscles of the neck be gently stretched on a daily basis. A physical therapist can help with exercises specifically for torticollis.

Best Acupressure Point for Torticollis
SI3 • Houxi (see Small Intestine 3, page 48)

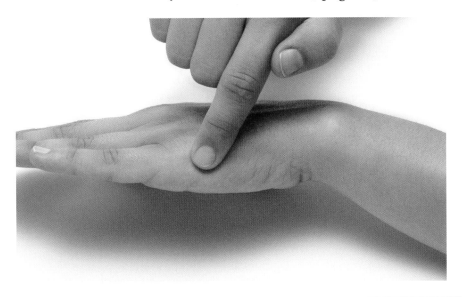

Other Acupressure Points to Consider

After pressing the best acupressure point for this condition, follow with one of these points:

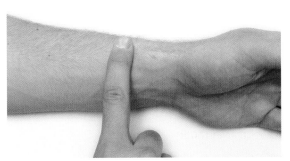

Also add LU7 • Lieque (see Lung 7, page 25)

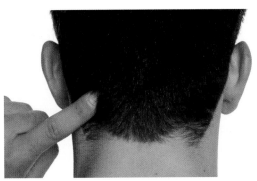

For torticollis with stiff neck, add GB20 • Fengchi (see Gallbladder 20, page 69) if the pain is in the scalenes on the side of the neck

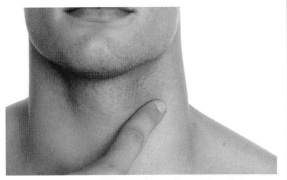

For torticollis with stiff neck, add ST9 • Renying (see Stomach 9, page 37) if the pain is in the sternocleidomastoid muscle (SCM) on the front of the neck

Trigeminal Neuralgia (Facial Nerve Pain)

Trigeminal neuralgia, also called tic douloureux, is pain of the trigeminal nerve. The nerve is responsible for relaying sensory information from the face to the brain. It also plays a role in our ability to chew. It's named for its three branches: the ophthalmic, carrying sensory information from areas of the eye; and the maxillary and mandibular, serving the upper and lower jaw respectively. The condition is usually brought on by changes in the blood vessels with age, leading to friction, which eventually impairs the function of the nerve.

Signs and Symptoms

Trigeminal neuralgia can manifest as pain in any area of the face served by the trigeminal nerve. Typically, this is shooting pain with an accompanying electric sensation. The pain is extreme, and the slightest touch can bring on symptoms.

The condition is rarely seen in young people as it is a type of degenerative disease.

Other Treatments

- Warming, moving foods like cayenne, ginger, black pepper, turmeric
- B vitamins, especially B12
- Essential fatty acids like those found in flax, hemp and fish oils

Aromatherapy for Acupoints

Vetiver on ST43

Subacute trigeminal neuralgia: pain blend (see page 136) on ST7

Severe pain: helichrysum in St. John's wort oil base on TW21 (Pain can be intense, so press only if you can tolerate it. Otherwise, just carefully apply a drop of the essential oil blend.)

Best Acupressure Point for Trigeminal Neuralgia

ST43 • Xiangu (see Stomach 43, page 41)

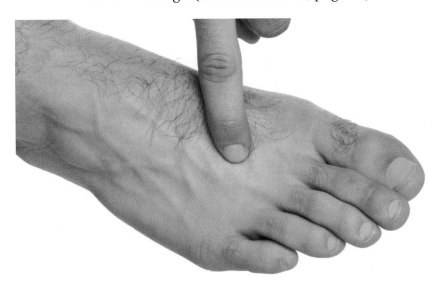

Other Acupressure Points to Consider

After pressing the best acupressure point for this condition, follow with one of these points:

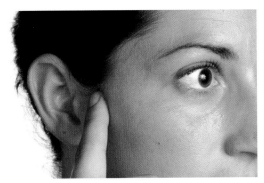

For subacute trigeminal neuralgia, add ST7 • Xiaguan (see Stomach 7, page 35)

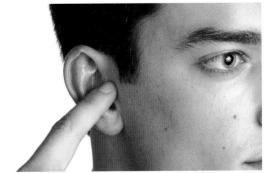

For trigeminal neuralgia with severe pain, add TW21 • Ermen (see Triple Warmer 21, page 65)

Ulcer

Ulcerations can occur anywhere along the entire length of the gastrointestinal tract. Most common are peptic ulcers, an inflammatory condition of the duodenum. Stomach ulcers are an inflammatory condition of the lining of the stomach. Esophageal ulcers occur less frequently, and ulcers of the colon occur in ulcerative colitis. The inflammation leads to the deterioration of the lining, resulting in holes, or ulcerations.

Stress used to be considered the main cause, but the spirochete-form bacterium *Helicobacter pylori* now fills that role, as it is present in up to 90% of cases (although studies seem to indicate this may be changing in some countries). *H. pylori* infections are diagnosed with a urea breath test and are relatively easy to treat with both conventional and natural medicine.

Patients who overuse certain pain medications may also experience ulcers.

Signs and Symptoms

Dull or burning pain is the primary symptom, often accompanied by heartburn or gastroesophageal reflux disease (GERD; see page 192). There may be an inability to tolerate certain foods high in fats, and alcohol, caffeine and cigarette smoking may exacerbate an existing ulcer. Queasiness or nausea are often present.

For those that have had an ulcer for some time, later symptoms may include vomiting blood. This is called "coffee ground" vomit because of its appearance, and may indicate other diseases as well. It is especially common with many liver diseases.

Aromatherapy for Acupoints

Mastic on ST36

With burning: chamomile on LI11

With sensations of cold in the stomach: ginger on SP4

With acid: orange on CV12

With dull ache: frankincense on PC7

> ### Note
> If an ulcer is bleeding (blood or black coloration in the stool or vomit that is bloody or looks like coffee grounds), seek immediate medical attention.

Other Treatments
- Orange peel tea (see box on page 192)
- D-limonene capsules are a more concentrated version if the tea does not help

Best Acupressure Point For Ulcer

ST36 • Zusanli (see Stomach 36, page 39)

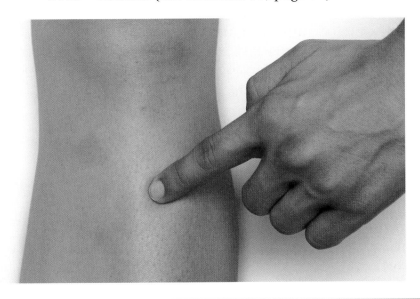

Other Acupressure Points to Consider

After pressing the best acupressure point for this condition, follow with one of these points:

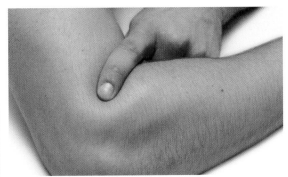

For ulcer with burning, add
LI11 • Quchi (see Large Intestine 11,
page 31)

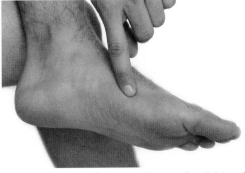

For ulcer with sensations of cold in the
stomach, add SP4 • Gongsun (see Spleen 4,
page 42)

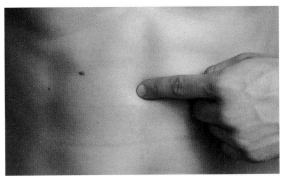

For ulcer with acid, add CV12 • Zhongwan
(see Conception Vessel 12, page 80)

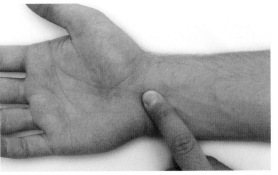

For ulcer with dull ache, add
PC7 • Daling (see Pericardium 7, page 62)

Urinary Incontinence

Urinary incontinence is an increasing difficulty with keeping urine in the bladder. The condition has many causes: age, surgery, nerve damage, lack of tone (not enough exercise), obesity, pregnancy and childbirth, age, stress and urinary tract infections. As the bladder is controlled by parasympathetic branches of the lower spinal nerves, an injury to the back could result in incontinence. Cystitis, bladder and kidney infections all have incontinence as a symptom.

Signs and Symptoms

Incontinence that occurs with age or injury is usually painless, but if there is an infection, burning and pain upon urination is common. Incontinence often begins with small leaks when laughing, coughing or sneezing, and it becomes more difficult to stop the flow in midstream.

Note
If incontinence comes on suddenly or is accompanied by persistent numbness or tingling, it could be a sign of a more serious condition and should be diagnosed by a doctor.

Other Treatments
- Exercises that strengthen the pelvic floor, such as Kegel exercises, may help
- Avoid triggers, such as alcohol, caffeine, sugar and spicy foods, that may worsen the situation
- Herb capsules that may help include bladderwrack, horsetail, saw palmetto, St. John's wort and marshmallow root

Strengthening the Pelvic Floor
Intentionally stopping the urine stream mid-flow can help reprogram the nerves and muscles that govern the sphincters, one of the muscles that control urine flow.

Aromatherapy for Acupoints

Carrot seed on CV4

With burning: blue chamomile on LR3

With prolapse: helichrysum on SP6

Best Acupressure Point for Urinary Incontinence

CV4 • Guanyuan (see Conception Vessel 4, page 78)

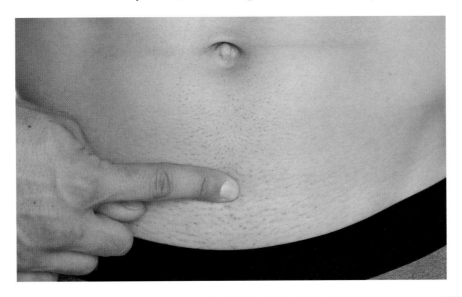

Other Acupressure Points to Consider

After pressing the best acupressure point for this condition, follow with one of these points:

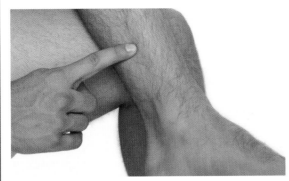

For urinary incontinence due to prolapse, add SP6 • Sanyinjiao (see Spleen 6, page 43)

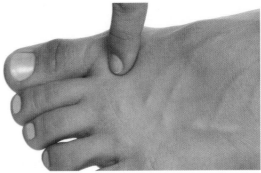

For urinary incontinence with burning, add LR3 • Taichong (see Liver 3, page 74)

Varicosities (Varicose Veins), Hemorrhoids

Weakened veins lead to a ballooning of the wall, seen externally as varicose veins or hemorrhoids. They can also occur around the belly button, on the abdomen or elsewhere in the body.

Unlike arteries, which have their own muscles to help them pump, the veins rely on physical movements of the body to move blood against gravity. Internal flaps work to hold the blood and prevent it from responding to gravity's pull.

Varicosities are seen when the flaps inside the veins stop functioning correctly. They become weak from inactivity or as a result of high blood pressure. Congenital weakness may be a factor, as can obesity and a sedentary lifestyle, or jobs that require a lot of standing, especially in one place, like hairdressing.

Some varicosities may be the result of straining, especially with constipation, but they can also result from a wracking cough or any condition that leads to increased pressure in the system. Vulvar varicosities can occur in pregnancy — moms can produce up to double the normal blood volume, putting increased pressure on the veins.

Signs and Symptoms

When the flaps in the deep veins fail, the blood flows back down into the vein, creating back pressure that results in convoluted, or "tortuous," veins at the skin surface. Burning or aching pain is common, and there may be itching, especially at the early stages.

Note

Gastric and esophageal varices are internal conditions leading to hidden bleeding. These can be very dangerous, life-threatening situations. The suggestions here are intended to help reduce the symptoms of varicose veins and hemorrhoids.

Other Treatments

- Try alternating hot and cold hydrotherapy
- If required to stand for long periods, try to change position and stretch the legs as often as possible
- Exercise in a water bath or pool to relieve the body of its own weight and help with venous return
- Horse chestnut, butcher's broom and ginkgo herbs help circulation
- To treat veins, apply Vein Blend (see box)

Aromatherapy for Acupoints

Spider veins: vein blend (see box) on SP10 and SP6

Hemorrhoids inserts: apply a cotton round moistened with witch hazel on CV1, or make your own suppositories with peppermint, cypress and St. John's wort oil for the pain (see page 230)

Varicosities of the vulva: Cypress on GV20. Also make your own salve with peppermint, cypress and St. John's wort oil for application at the site of the varicosities.

Vein Blend

Add 2 drops each of carrot seed, helichrysum and cypress essential oils to 1 ounce (30 mL) of calophyllum inophyllum (tamanu) fixed oil.

Best Acupressure Point for Varicosities

SP10 • Xuehai (see Spleen 10, page 45)

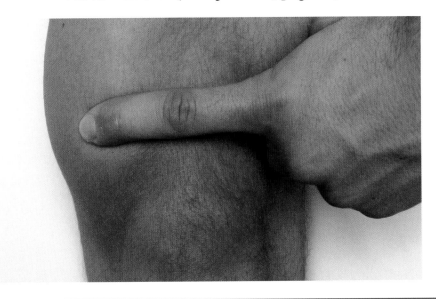

Other Acupressure Points to Consider

After pressing the best acupressure point for this condition, follow with one of these points:

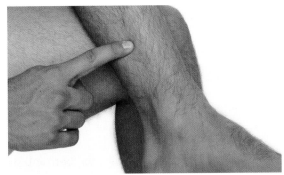

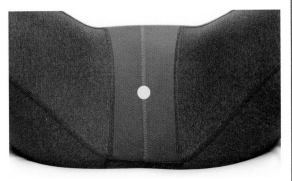

For varicose veins in legs, add
SP6 • Sanyinjiao (see Spleen 6, page 43)

For hemorrhoids, add CV1 • Huiyin
(see Conception Vessel 1, page 76)

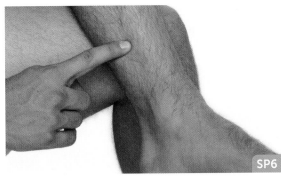

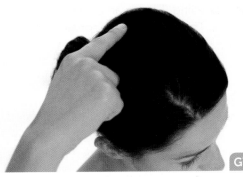

For vulvar varicosities, add SP6 • Sanyinjiao (see Spleen 6, page 43)
and GV20 • Baihui (see Governing Vessel 20, page 84)

Vertigo and Light-Headedness

Vertigo is the sensation that the room is spinning, or an internal sense of spinning, that often occurs upon moving from sitting to standing but can occur any time. Vertigo is common in the elderly, either due to poor circulation or from drug interactions. The condition may be a sign of an inner ear problem, as the otoliths (bony structures in the ear) are partly responsible for our sense of balance. Some conditions, such as Ménière's disease or migraine headaches, have vertigo as a symptom. Head injuries may also result in vertigo.

Light-headedness is the sensation of feeling faint or weak with no sense that the surroundings are moving. Feeling light-headed can happen anytime and may have many different causes. Illness often causes the sensation. Changes in blood sugar, hunger, starvation and dehydration can all lead to feeling light-headed. Many medications warn of light-headedness as a side effect.

Signs and Symptoms

Dizziness is the main symptom of vertigo. Light-headedness describes the main symptom. There may also be a feeling of weakness, sometimes so strong there is a need to sit immediately. Sweating and clamminess also often occur. There may be brain fog or confusion for a few seconds. With vertigo, falling is a real concern. The sensation that everything is moving is very disconcerting, leading to mental confusion. It may result in nausea and vomiting.

Note

In some cases, vertigo may indicate a more serious condition. If the condition does not improve or worsens, consider seeing a doctor.

Other Treatments

- CoQ10 may be helpful to regulate blood (and qi) flow to the head
- Ginkgo and butcher's broom help with poor circulation

Aromatherapy for Acupoints

Upon standing (not enough qi moving up to the head): rosemary or cinnamon on GV20

With throbbing in the head (too much qi moving up to the head): cypress or cedarwood on GB43

With a feeling of floating out of the body: vetiver on KI1

Best Acupressure Point for Vertigo and Light-Headedness

GV20 • Baihui (see Governing Vessel 20, page 84)

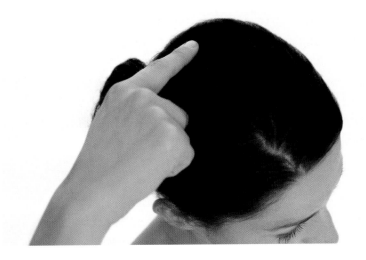

Other Acupressure Points to Consider

After pressing the best acupressure point for this condition, follow with one of these points:

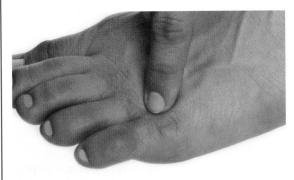

For vertigo with throbbing in the head (too much qi moving up to the head), add GB43 • Xiaxi (see Gallbladder 43, page 72)

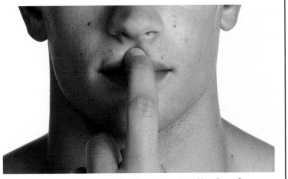

For vertigo with that typically leads to fainting, add GV26 • Shuigou (see Governing Vessel 26, page 85)

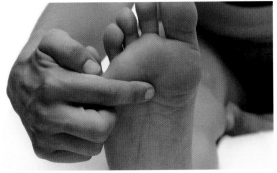

For vertigo with a feeling of floating out of the body, add KI1 • Yongquan (see Kidney 1, page 54)

Viral Infections

Viruses can cause many different kinds of infections, from the common cold and influenza to chickenpox, gastroenteritis or herpes. Some very dangerous conditions, such as Ebola and hantavirus infection, are viral, but fortunately these conditions are more rare.

Signs and Symptoms

Each viral infection will manifest with its own set of symptoms. The most common viral conditions are:

- Childhood illnesses: measles, mumps, rubella
- Respiratory: flu (influenza), pneumonia, sinusitis
- Gastrointestinal: gastroenteritis
- Skin: chickenpox, shingles, warts
- Nervous system: encephalitis, meningitis
- Reproductive: genital warts, genital herpes
- Liver: hepatitis

Many viral infections are serious. Each will have specific cautions based on the virus and the health of the individual. The suggestions here are to help reduce symptoms and inhibit viral growth by making changes to strengthen the internal milieu.

Other Treatments

- For sore throat, see page 240; for hepatitis and liver disease, see page 198
- Diffuse lemon and eucalyptus into sick rooms; use personal warm (not hot!) steam inhalation with the same for all infections
- Clean surfaces. Many viruses can live on surfaces for long periods of time
- Rest as much as possible
- For cold sores, use Lysine, applied topically and taken internally
- For gastroenteritis, take thyme or oregano capsules
- Consider these supplements: reishi mushroom, echinacea, vitamin C, melissa capsules and cat's claw

Healing Bone Broth

For all viral infections, it's important to stay hydrated. For greater healing, drink a good-quality vegetable or bone broth made with garlic and onion and sip as a soup. Adding cayenne and parsley will give it an extra boost.

Aromatherapy for Acupoints

Systemic: eucalyptus globulus on LI11; for kids, eucalyptus radiata on LI4

Affecting the respiratory: Ravintsara on LU9

Affecting the reproductive: thyme on LR8

Affecting the gastrointestinal: myrrh on CV12

Affecting the liver: carrot seed and eucalyptus citriodora on LR3

Cold sores: melissa on ST7

Best Acupressure Point for Viral Infections

LI11 • Quchi (see Large Intestine 11, page 31)

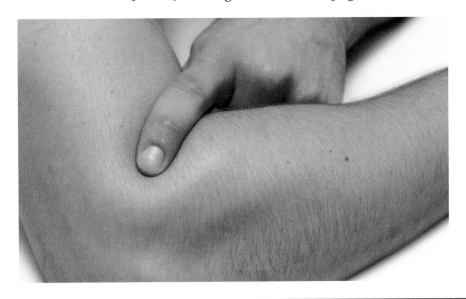

Other Acupressure Points to Consider

After pressing the best acupressure point for this condition, follow with one of these points:

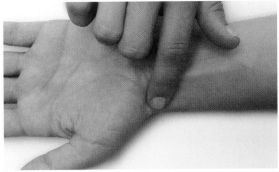

For viral infections affecting the respiratory system, add LU9 • Taiyuan (see Lung 9, page 26)

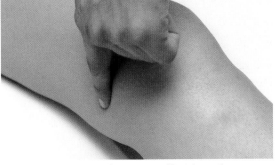

For viral infections affecting the reproductive system, add LR8 • Ququan (see Liver 8, page 75)

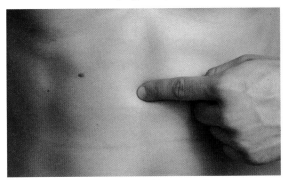

For viral infections affecting the gastro-intestinal tract, add CV12 • Zhongwan (see Conception Vessel 12, page 80)

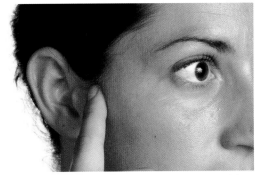

For viral infections with cold sores, add ST7 • Xiaguan (see Stomach 7, page 35)

Glossary

Aldehyde: an oxygenated compound found in many essential oils

Anesthetizing: reduces sensation

Antalgic: reduces back pain

Anti-infective agent: an agent a substance capable of acting against infection

Anti-inflammatory: reduces inflammation

Antiallergenic: reduces the likelihood of an allergic response

Antibacterial: reduces bacterial load

Anticatarrhal: helps remove stubborn, thickened mucus from the body

Anticoagulant: decreases coagulation of the blood

Antifungal: deters the growth of fungus

Antihistamine: reduces the receptivity of the histamine receptors and thus the levels of histamine released

Antihypercholesterolemic agent: reduces elevated serum cholesterol levels

Antihypertensive: reduces hypertension (high blood pressure) and its symptoms

Antiparasitic: reduces parasites

Antipruritic: stops itch

Antipyretic: has a cooling effect

Antirheumatic: reduces symptoms of or delays the progression of rheumatic diseases (inflammatory conditions of the connective tissue)

Antiseptic: inhibits the growth of microorganisms

Antispasmodic: reduces spasms

Antiviral: reduces viral loads or discourages the proliferation of viruses

Aphrodisiac: arouses sexual desire

Appetite stimulant: increases appetite

Ascaris species: a parasitic roundworm

Atherosclerotic plaques: a substance built up of cholesterol and blood factors that leads to a narrowing of the blood vessels

Bacteriocidal: a substance capable of killing bacteria

Biochemical: the chemical processes of living organisms

Bioenergetic: the energetic processes of living organisms

CNS depressant: reduces hyperactivity in the central nervous system (brain and spinal cord)

Candida albicans: a fungal agent responsible for opportunistic fungal infections such as thrush

Cardiac tonic: tones the tissues of the heart

Carminative: reduces the production of gas in the gastrointestinal system

Cell-regenerating: encourages the proliferation of new cells

Cholagogue: promotes the production and discharge of bile

Choleretic: substances that increase the production of bile

Cicatrisant: an agent that causes a wound to heal or become healed by the formation of scar tissue

Cortisone-like: functions like naturally occurring cortisone

Cough suppressant: stops cough

Cytochrome P450 liver detoxification: the enzyme system used by the liver to metabolize and clear substances

Decongestant: reduces congestion in tissues and organs

Detoxifying: helps remove stored toxins from the body; may encourage the cytochrome P450 liver detoxification cycle

Digestive enzymes: substances that help break down food

Digestive tonic: tones organs of digestion

Diuretic: removes excess fluids from the body by promoting the production of urine

Douche: a medicinal liquid delivered into the vagina via a bottle or bag

Edema: pathological accumulation of fluids in various parts of the body

Endocrine tonic: tones the glands of the endocrine system

Emmenagogue: stimulates blood flow in the pelvis and uterus

Enema: a medicinal liquid delivered into the anus via a bottle or bag

Estrogen-like: functions like naturally occurring estrogen

Expectorant: helps the lungs expel mucus

Febrifuge: helps reduce a fever

Galactogogue: encourages the production of breast milk

Hemostatic: helps slow or stop the flow of blood

Hepatic activity: activity of or relating to the liver

Hepatoregenerative: encourages the regeneration of liver cells

Hepatostimulant: stimulates activity in the liver

Homeodynamics: the constantly changing interrelatedness of all components within a system as they attempt to maintain overall equilibrium

Hormone-like: acts like naturally occurring hormones

Hyperactive pain response: a heightened reaction to pain, either in frequency or intensity

Hypertensive: may increase blood pressure

Insectifuge: drives away insects

Lipolytic: causes lipolysis, the breakdown of fatty substances

Litholitic: helps dissolve calculi (stones) in the body

Lymphatic decongestant: decreases congestion of the lymphatic system

Microbials: agents that kill or decrease bacteria

Microcirculation: the circulation occurring in the capillaries, usually at the periphery

Monoterpene: a hydrocarbon made up of two isoprene units; found in many essential oils

Mucolytic: liquifies and moves thick mucus. May increase thin mucus that aids in the expectoration of thick, sticky mucus

Muscular contracture: a state of temporary or permanent tension in a muscle that leads to decreased function

Mycobactericidal: a substance capable of killing Mycobacterium, the microbe responsible for diseases such as tuberculosis and leprosy

Nervous system–regulating: balances the nervous system

Nervous system tonic: tones the nervous system

Neuroregulatory effects: help regulate neurological activity; for example, reduce hyperactivity or increase focus

Neurotonic: tones brain function

Parasympathetic nervous system: part of the autonomic nervous system responsible for reducing sympathetic responses; primarily it helps put the body into the rest phase

Peripheral neuropathies: malfunctions of the nerves carrying messages from the extremities

Pessary: another word for suppository, although pessaries are often delivered via a device that helps support internal structures, for example, a prolapse

Preservative: slows degeneration and breakdown

Regulates cardiac rhythm: helps balance heart rate and rhythm

Remodels scar tissue: dissolves scars and encourages new skin

Respiratory tonic: tones the respiratory system

Rheumatic diseases: inflammatory conditions of the connective tissue

Staph species: staphylococcus species bacteria, responsible for many bacterial infections, including methicillin-resistant Staphyloccus aureus (MRSA)

Sedative: encourages calm, relaxation and sleep

Strep species: a streptococcus species; the bacterial agent responsible for many diseases, such as meningitis and strep throat

Styptic: a substance that arrests bleeding

Sudoriferous glands: sweat glands

Suppository: a therapeutic preparation in solid form designed to be inserted into the vagina or anus. Suppositories slowly melt and deliver their benefits over time.

Sympathetic nervous system: part of the autonomic nervous system that increases sympathetic responses; that is, the functions that allow the body to respond to stressors

Thermoreceptors: the part of a sensory neuron that detects temperature and temperature changes

Thyroid tonic: tones the thyroid gland

Varicosities: weakness in the wall of a vein that leads to ballooning and reduced function

Vasodilatory: dilates blood vessels to decrease pressure

Venous: of or relating to the system of veins

Venous decongestant: reduces congestion in the veins

Vermicidal: a substance that kills worms

Vermifuge: a substance that changes the internal milieu to be inhospitable to parasitic worms or actively kills parasitic worms

Virucidal: capable of killing viruses

Vulnerary: assists in wound healing

Wide-spectrum antibiotic: an agent capable of killing a broad range of life forms

References

Articles

Antibiotic, Antifungal, Anti-inflammatory

Boukhatem M, Ferhat M, Kameli A, Saidi F, Kebir H. Lemon grass (*Cymbopogon citratus*) essential oil as a potent anti-inflammatory and antifungal drugs. *Libyan J Med*, 2014 Sep; 9: 25431.

Gbenou J, Ahounou J, Akakpo H, Laleye A, Yayi E, Gbaguidi F, Baba-Moussa L, Darboux R, Dansou P, Moudachirou M, Kotchoni S. Phytochemical composition of *Cymbopogon citratus* and *Eucalyptus citriodora* essential oils and their anti-inflammatory and analgesic properties on Wistar rats. *Mol Biol Rep*, 2013 Feb; 40(2): 1127–34.

Husain S, Ali M. Volatile oil constituents of the leaves of *Eucalyptus citriodora* and influence on clinically isolated pathogenic microorganisms. *J Sci Inno Res,* 2013 2(5): 852–58.

Maruzzella J, Liguori.L. The in vitro antifungal activity of essential oils. *J Am Pharm Assoc*, 1958 Apr; 47(4): 250–54.

Pattnaik S, Subramanyam V, Kole C. Antibacterial and antifungal activity of ten essential oils in vitro. *Microbios*, 1996; 86(349): 237–46.

Russell W, Duthie G. Plant secondary metabolites and gut health: the case for phenolic acids. *Proc Nutr Soc*, 2011 Aug; 70(3): 389–96.

Anxiety, Depression

Setzer W. Essential oils and anxiolytic aromatherapy, 2009 Sep; 4(9): 1305-16.

WebMD. Drugs that cause depression. Available at: www.webmd.com/depression/guide./medicines-cause-depression?page=2

Alopecia (Hair Loss)

Lanomache L, Benea V. Stress in patients with alopecia areata and vitiligo. *J Eur Acad Dermatol*, 2007 Aug; 21(7): 921–28

Breastfeeding

Lemay D, Ballard O, Hughes M, Morrow A, Horseman N, Rivers L. RNA sequencing of the human milk fat layer transcriptome reveals distinct gene expression profiles at three stages of lactation. *PLoS One*, 2013 July; 8(7): e67531.

Cinnamon

Sartorius T, Peter A, Schulz N, Drescher A,Bergheim I, Machann J, Schick F, Siegel-Axel D, Schürmann A, Weigert C, Häring H-U, Hennige A. Cinnamon extract improves insulin sensitivity in the brain and lowers liver fat in mouse models of obesity. *PLoS One*, 2014 March; 9(3): e92358.

Ginger

Ghayur M, Gilani A. Inhibitory activity of ginger rhizome on airway and uterine smooth muscle preparations. *Eur Food Res Technol*, 2007 Jan; 224(4): 477–81.

Vutyavanich T, Kraisarin T, Ruangsri R. Ginger for nausea and vomiting in pregnancy: randomized, double-masked, placebo-controlled trial. *Obstet Gynecol*, 2001 Apr; 97(4): 577–82.

Gastroprotective

Testerman T, Morris J. Beyond the stomach: An updated view of *Helicobacter pylori* pathogenesis, diagnosis, and treatment. *World J Gastroenterol*, 2014 Sep; 20(36): 12781–808.

Tilg H, Kaser A. Diet and relapsing ulcerative colitis: take off the meat? *Gut*, 2004 Oct; 53(10): 1399–1401.

Hygiene Hypothesis

Shi J, Liu YL, Fang YX, Xu GZ, Zhai HF, Lu L. Traditional Chinese medicine in treatment of opiate addiction. *Acta Pharmacol Sin*, 2006 Oct; 27(10): 1303–08.

Sun J. D-limonene: safety and clinical applications. *Altern Med Rev*, 2007 Sep; 12(3): 259–64.

Tinnitus (Ringing in the Ears)

von Boetticher A. *Ginkgo biloba* extract in the treatment of tinnitus: a systematic review. *Neuropsychiatr Dis Treat*, 2011 July; 7: 441–47.

Okada D, Onishi E, Chami F, Borin A, Cassola N, Guerreiro V. Acupuncture for tinnitus immediate relief. *Braz J Otorhinolaryngol*, 2006 Mar–Apr; 72(2): 182–06.

Books

Clarke S. *Essential Chemistry for Aromatherapy*. 2nd ed. Edinburgh, UK: Churchill Livingstone; 2009.

Herrera M. *Holy Smoke: The Use of Incense in the Catholic Church*. 2nd ed. San Luis Obispo, CA: Tixlini Scriptorium; 2012.

Forbes R. (1970). *A Short History of the Art of Distillation: From the Beginnings up to the Death of Cellier Blumenthal*. Leiden, Netherlands: Brill; 1970.

Franchomme P, Jollois R, Pénoël D. *L'Aromathérapie exactemente: Encyclopedie, de l'utilisation therapeutique des huiles essentielles.* Paris, France: Roger Jollois; 2001.

Haw, G.S. *Marco Polo in China: A Venetian in the Realm of Khubilai Khan.* London, UK: Routledge; 2006: 147–48.

Keville K, Green M. *Aromatherapy: A Complete Guide to the Healing Art.* Berkeley, CA: Crossing Press; 1995.

Schnaubelt K. *Advanced Aromatherapy: The Science of Essential Oil Therapy.* Rochester, VT: Healing Arts; 1998.

Stoddart D. *The Scented Ape: The Biology and Culture of Human Odour.* Cambridge, UK: Cambridge University Press; 1990.

Tisserand R, Young R. *Essential Oil Safety: A Guide for Health Professionals.* 2nd ed. Edinburgh, UK: Churchill Livingstone; 2013.

Willmont D. *Aromatherapy with Chinese Medicine: Healing the Body/Mind/Spirit with Essential Oils.* Marshfield, MA: Willmountain; 2003.

Yuen J. *Materia Medica of Essential Oils: Based on a Chinese Medical Perspective.* Los Angeles, CA: Lotus Center for Integrative Medicine, 2000.

Essential Websites

Dr. Heiner Fruehauf's work can be found at www.classicalchinesemedicine.org

Luminous Presence
luminouspresencepdx.com

National Association for Holistic Aromatherapy
naha.org

Robert Tisserand
roberttisserand.com

Snow Lotus:
Aromatherapy, Education, Inspiration
snowlotus.org

ESSENTIAL OIL RETAILERS:

Floracopeia
floracopeia.com

Original Swiss Aromatics
originalswissaromatics.com

Veriditas By Pranarom
veriditasbotanicals.com

Index

nettle tea, 138, 204
nettles, 208, 210, 230, 234
niacin, 142
niaouli *(Melaleuca quinquenervia)*, **120,** 190
nicotine addiction, 116, 134, 135
nocturnal enuresis, 43, 55, 112, 121, 123, 125, **224–225**
nose, 57
  see also runny nose; stuffy nose
nosebleed, 28, 29, 33, 53, 55, 85
NSAIDs, 186
numbness, 64, 70, 236, 237

O

oil pulling, 146, 194, 246
okra, 174, 240
omega-3 fatty acids, 148, 238
onion skin broth, 138
onions, 162
opiates, 180
oral ingestion, 101–102
orange *(Citrus aurantium),* 102, **120,** 168, 170, 178, 184, 192, 202, 206, 242, 252
orange peel tea, 192, 252
order, 92–94
oregano *(Origanum vulgare),* **121,** 127, 154, 184, 212, 224, 230, 260
osteoarthritis, 111, 117, 148
over-the-counter laxatives, 174
oxygenated hydrocarbons, 106

P

pain, 110, 115, 116, 126, 196
  see also specific types of pain
pain blend, 136, 148, 166, 188, 212, 214, 228, 232, 236, 248, 250
painful cough, 27
palpitations, 59, 62
panic attacks, 144
passionflower, 206
patchouli *(Pogostemon cablin),* **121,** 190, 238
patterns
  disruption of natural patterns, 11–12
  greater patterns, 13–16
PC6. *See* Pericardium 6 (PC6, Neiguan)
PC7. *See* Pericardium 7 (PC7, Daling)
pelvic floor, 254
pelvic inflammatory disease, 210
Penoel, Daniel, 104
peppermint *(Mentha piperita),* 101, 102, **121,** 127, 158, 160, 170, 176, 190, 192, 196, 200, 220, 222, 226, 230, 234, 246, 256
Pericardium 6 (PC6, Neiguan), **61,** 134, 135, 142, 143, 144, 145, 156, 157, 158, 159, 192, 193, 207, 220, 221, 222, 223
Pericardium 7 (PC7, Daling), **62,** 166, 167, 252, 253
pessary, 101

pharyngitis, 240
phenols, 106, 107, 184
phlegm, 26, 40, 46, 59, 60, 110, 113, 114, 115, 117, 121, 122, 124, 162, **226–227**
phobia, 144
photosensitizing, 105
pine *(Pinus sylvestris),* **122,** 144, 176, 226, 240, 242
pinkeye. *See* conjunctivitis (pinkeye)
placenta, retained, 53, 77
plantar fasciitis, 54, 116, 118, 119, 123, **228–229**
plastics, 11
pneumocystis pneumonia, 190
pneumonia, 194
polycystic ovary syndrome, 210
postnasal drip, 194
postpartum imbalances, 46
potassium, 186
pregnancy and childbirth
  acupressure points to avoid, 29, 38, 43, 53, 77, 78, 79
  anemia in postpartum, 45
  delivery in childbirth, 29
  ectopic pregnancies, 210
  essential oils, 105
  gestational diabetes, 182
  labor, encouragement of, 53
  morning sickness, 61, 220–221
  placenta, retained, 53, 77
  plantar fasciitis, 228
  postpartum imbalances, 46
  retained placenta, 53
preventive bedwetting drink, 224
probiotics, 174, 194, 202, 222
prolapse, 178, 179, 255
  see also specific types of prolapse
pronation, 228, 229
prostate cancer, 160
prostate infections, 73, 76
prostatitis, 73, 76, 115, 121, 125, **230–231**
pumpkin, 186, 218
pumpkin seeds, 230
purpose, lack of, 58
purslane, 240

Q

qi, 11, 20, 21, 96, 108, 130
qigong, 224
Quchi. *See* Large Intestine 11 (LI11, Quchi)
quercetin, 138, 164, 234
Ququan. *See* Liver 8 (LR8, Ququan)

R

raspberry leaves, 204
ratio of yin and yang, 13
Ravintsara *(Cinnamomum camphora),* **122,** 127, 162, 170, 176, 240, 260
raw honey, 176, 224
Raynaud syndrome, 26, 46, 111, 116, 122, 123, **232–233**

rectal prolapse (protrusion), 50, 84, 161
rectal suppository, 230
red clover, 204, 210, 218
reishi mushroom, 260
Renying. *See* Stomach 9 (ST9, Renying)
repair salve, 152
reproductive imbalances, 43
reproductive organs, conditions of, 76
reproductive system, 260, 261
respiratory conditions, 131, 162
  see also specific respiratory conditions
respiratory fungal infections, 190
respiratory system, 260, 261
respiratory viral infections, 122
rest and digest, 222
restlessness, 87
retained placenta, 53
rheumatoid arthritis, 113, 148
rhinitis, 33, 110, 111, 115, 116, 117, 121, 123, **234–235**
ringing in the ears. *See* tinnitus
Roman chamomile *(Anthemis nobilis),* **111,** 127, 148, 150, 200, 208, 232
rose, 142, 144, 156, 164, 180, 206, 212, 216, 218, 232, 238, 246
rose geranium. *See* geranium, rose *(Pelargonium graveolens)*
rose hip seed, 146
rose otto *(Rosa damascena),* **122,** 127
rose sandalwood, 162
rosemary *(Rosemarinus officinalis),* 101, **123,** 127, 136, 140, 142, 150, 176, 182, 204, 210, 224, 228, 230, 232, 234, 236, 258
rosemary verbenone, 140, 184, 238
runny nose, 25, 33, 85, 110, 111, 115, 116, 117, 121, 123, **234–235**

S

sage *(Salvia officinalis),* **123,** 234
salivation, 83
SAM-e (S-adenosylmethionine), 180
sandalwood, 144, 212, 218
Sanyinjiao. *See* Spleen 6 (SP6, Sanyinjiao)
saw palmetto, 230, 254
Schnaubelt, Kurt, 104
sciatica, 70, 71, 110, 116, 123, **236–237**
scullcap, 206
seasonal affective disorder (SAD), 180
seaweed, 242
seizure disorder, 105
selenium, 230, 238
self-care, 12
seminal emissions, 55
sensitization, 102
sensory organs, 30, 48
sesquiterpenes, 106
sesquiterpenols, 107

Library and Archives Canada Cataloguing in Publication

Parramore, Karin, 1964-, author
    The essential step-by-step guide to acupressure with aromatherapy : relief for 64 common health conditions / Karin Parramore, LAC, CH.

Includes index.
ISBN 978-0-7788-0546-5 (paperback)

    1. Acupressure. 2. Aromatherapy. I. Title.

RM723.A27P37 2016   615.8'222   C2016-905299-0